Better Homes and Gardens®

EAT&STAY SLIM

© Copyright 1979 by Meredith Corporation, Des Moines, Iowa.
All Rights Reserved. Printed in the United States of America.
Large-Format Edition. Seventh Printing, 1985.
Library of Congress Catalog Card Number: 78-74939
ISBN: 0-696-01115-8

BETTER HOMES AND GARDENS® BOOKS
Editor-in-Chief: James A. Autry
Editorial Director: Neil Kuehnl
Executive Art Director: William J. Yates

Editor: Gerald M. Knox
Art Director: Ernest Shelton
Associate Art Directors: Randall Yontz,
    Neoma Alt West
Copy and Production Editors: David Kirchner, Lamont Olson,
    David A. Walsh
Assistant Art Director: Harijs Priekulis
Senior Graphic Designer: Faith Berven
Graphic Designers: Linda Ford, Richard Lewis,
    Sheryl Veenschoten, Tom Wegner,

Food Editor: Doris Eby
Senior Associate Food Editor: Sharyl Heiken
Senior Food Editors: Sandra Granseth, Elizabeth Woolever
Associate Food Editors: Mary Cunningham, Joanne Johnson,
    Joy Taylor, Pat Teberg
Recipe Development Editor: Marion Viall
Test Kitchen Director: Sharon Golbert
Test Kitchen Home Economists: Jean Brekke, Kay Cargill,
    Marilyn Cornelius, Maryellyn Krantz, Marge Steenson

Eat and Stay Slim
Editors: Joanne Johnson, Sandra Granseth
Consultant: Pat Jester, Creative Foods Limited
Medical Consultant: Philip L. White, Sc.D., Director, Department
    of Foods and Nutrition, American Medical Association
Copy and Production Editor: Lamont Olson
Graphic Designer: Sheryl Veenschoten

On the cover: Eat all these foods in one day and still lose weight (see page 45 for menu). Recipes for the 1,200-calorie Daily Meal Plan, clockwise from back, are: Mexican-Style Hot Chocolate (see recipe, page 52); Tapioca Pudding Parfait (see recipe, page 80); Taco Compuesto (see recipe, page 59); Turkey Asparagus Stacks (see recipe, page 69); Herbed Tomato Soup (see recipe, page 55); and Pineapple Dream Pie (see recipe, page 76).

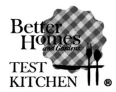

Our seal assures you that every recipe in *Eat and Stay Slim* is endorsed by the Better Homes and Gardens Test Kitchen. Each recipe is tested for family appeal, practicality, and deliciousness.

contents

chapter 1

should you reduce?

Eat and stay slim. That may sound too good to be true, but it's not. Whether you're just thinking about losing weight, or already slim and trying to stay that way, the formula is simple: Eat tasty, nutritious meals and enjoy every bite. With our system of weight control, years of eating and staying slim lie ahead of you.

If you are more than 15 pounds overweight, ask your doctor whether you should reduce (if he hasn't told you already). If he says to reduce, you should. No ifs or buts. Listen to medical advice.

Why go to a doctor about such an obvious problem as excess weight? Why not plunge into the latest fad diet without bothering your doctor? There are several good reasons.

Doctor's orders

The best reason for consulting a doctor is that a physical checkup will determine what ails you, if anything, besides your weight. The risks of hypertension, diabetes, gallbladder disease, joint disease aggravation, and cardiovascular disease increase as your degree of excess weight increases. Your doctor can check these things before you begin a reducing program.

Your doctor probably will advise you to avoid any fad diet that extols one or two foods, supposedly bursting with slimming "miracles." Some reducing diets push kelp or other sources of iodine that can produce signs of iodine toxicity in the body. Some diets stress one class of foods at the expense of others. This can result in omission of foods which provide essential nutrients. Diets excessively high in one nutrient—fats, proteins, carbohydrates —can just as easily be looked on as low in something else. Restrict your carbohydrate intake excessively and you'll likely be on a high-fat diet without knowing it. Do not attempt a starvation diet or protein-supplemented fast without close medical supervision. This book avoids that sort of thing; you eat, not starve, to slimness.

Weight control is not a matter of crash reducing for brief periods of time. It's a lifetime proposition and the foods you eat while reducing should be the kind that you would like to eat forever.

Believe it or not, a few people who are already beanpole slim want to reduce. A doctor can prevent such dangerous folly by giving them sound medical guidance.

Telltale bulges

To reduce safely you must have excess fat to lose. Generally, excess fat is all too visible. Stand naked in front of a full-length mirror. Look for telltale bulges, such as fleshy pads or "spare tires." Fat tends to cluster in slightly different areas in men and women.

Women: under chin, back of neck, breasts, abdomen, upper arms, buttocks, hips, thighs.

Men: under chin, back of neck, abdomen, trunk.

Stand erect, sink your chin into your chest, and look down. If you can't see your toes without craning your neck, you have something to lose.

Tense your abdominal muscles as if someone were aiming a blow at you. While doing this, press your fingertips over your midriff. If the fat pad over the muscles feels soft and cushiony, you could spare some of it. A physically fit person should be able to feel the hardness of tensed muscles and even see a muscular ripple or two.

The "pinch test" gives another clue to excess body fat. Stand straight and have someone pinch just below your shoulder blades or at the back of your upper arm. Is there fat to spare?

Do last year's clothes have shrinking fits? Have your waistline and neckline measurements increased in the last five years or so? If you're more than 25 years old, could you get into the same clothes you wore then? Has the width of your shoe size increased? Do buttons and zippers have that strained look?

Such signs may persuade you that you have fat to lose. Another way is to check your standing against a weight chart. Weight charts have the advantage of being completely impersonal and

objective. Standards of desirable weight are given on page 6. Weigh yourself without shoes and clothing, check the chart, and find out how you measure up to the desirable weight levels.

Normal weights in healthy persons will vary over a wide range because of individual differences in body structure. Persons with larger than average builds (wide shoulders and hips, large wrists and ankles) should weigh between the average and high figures given in the table on page 6. Persons with small builds (narrow shoulders and hips, small wrists and ankles) probably should weigh no more than the average and no less than the low figures given for their height. Most people, however, have medium or average frames. Frequently, an overweight person will use a weight table to justify the extra weight by claiming his or her frame is bigger than it really is. Chances are that if your weight exceeds your desirable weight by 10 pounds or more, your doctor will tell you it's time to reduce.

Occasionally, excess weight is not caused by excess fat. Large amounts of water (which weighs more than fat) may accumulate in body tissue and tip the scales. Abnormal water retention is usually associated with some physical disorder. That's just another reason why you should consult your doctor before you start a reducing program of any kind— to evaluate your overall health status.

Why reduce your weight?

Better personal appearance is a wonderful rea- son for keeping your weight normal, but there are other reasons. Obesity is frequently associated with high blood pressure and the onset of diabetes in susceptible persons. Excess fat makes breathing less efficient and puts a cruel and heavy load on joints that have to support it. Besides, overweight people usually will have shorter life spans. And an impediment to vitality is lifted when useless dead weight is removed from the vital organs.

If you've just discovered that you need to shed a few extra pounds, you're not alone. It has been estimated that at least half the adults in the United States are either overweight or obese. Pretty astounding, isn't it? With all the talk about fitness and diets, one would think that Americans are a slim bunch. Not so. As a group, Americans today are fatter than their counterparts a generation ago.

Many people manage to shed a few unwanted pounds. However, few people keep these pounds off. Once you've mastered our system of weight control, you can lose pounds and keep them off forever.

desirable weight levels

women

HEIGHT	LOW	AVERAGE	HIGH
60 inches	100 pounds	109 pounds	118 pounds
61 inches	104 pounds	112 pounds	121 pounds
62 inches	107 pounds	115 pounds	125 pounds
63 inches	110 pounds	118 pounds	128 pounds
64 inches	113 pounds	122 pounds	132 pounds
65 inches	116 pounds	125 pounds	135 pounds
66 inches	120 pounds	129 pounds	139 pounds
67 inches	123 pounds	132 pounds	142 pounds
68 inches	126 pounds	136 pounds	146 pounds
69 inches	130 pounds	140 pounds	151 pounds
70 inches	133 pounds	144 pounds	156 pounds
71 inches	137 pounds	148 pounds	161 pounds
72 inches	141 pounds	152 pounds	166 pounds

men

HEIGHT	LOW	AVERAGE	HIGH
63 inches	118 pounds	129 pounds	141 pounds
64 inches	122 pounds	133 pounds	145 pounds
65 inches	126 pounds	137 pounds	149 pounds
66 inches	130 pounds	142 pounds	155 pounds
67 inches	134 pounds	147 pounds	161 pounds
68 inches	139 pounds	151 pounds	166 pounds
69 inches	143 pounds	155 pounds	170 pounds
70 inches	147 pounds	159 pounds	174 pounds
71 inches	150 pounds	163 pounds	178 pounds
72 inches	154 pounds	167 pounds	183 pounds
73 inches	158 pounds	171 pounds	188 pounds
74 inches	162 pounds	175 pounds	192 pounds
75 inches	165 pounds	178 pounds	195 pounds

The measurements in this chart are without shoes or clothing.

how excess weight comes and goes

How does excess body fat pile up where it's not wanted?

It comes from eating more food than we burn up through physical activity and the bodily processes that require energy.

Here's the how of it: Foods furnish energy that is measured in heat units called calories. If we take in more calories from food and drink than we burn up through activity and basic body functions, the surplus calories are stashed away in the form of body fat. The body acts as a sort of fat bank. If excessive intake of calories continues, the fat bank bulges and bulges from the heavy deposits.

Reducing is a matter of making withdrawals from the fat bank. There are only two safe ways to do this: (1) eat less and reduce calorie intake; and/or (2) increase physical activity and burn up more calories. Either way, a calorie deficit results.

In short, reducing requires a low-calorie diet combined when possible with more activity to help you slim faster and feel better. That's what this book is about.

Automatic calorie counters

Your body never fails to count a calorie, even if you fail to. It's not necessary to look up calorie tables when you plan meals. It's much easier to let Food Exchanges count calories for you—a pleasant relief indeed.

As explained on page 16, Food Exchanges are units of the foods—meats, vegetables, fats, fruits, etc.—that are foundations of good nutrition. The Food Exchanges, long used by professional dietitians, furnish definite amounts of calories. So, in planning meals, Food Exchanges not only help balance the diet and allow personal choices of foods you like, but also count your calories automatically.

One thing about it: You're *sure* to shed excess fat if your calorie deficit is sufficient to make withdrawals from your fat bank. It's also well to remember that everything that makes fat enters via the mouth. That's where fat control begins. And all too often that's where it ends.

When extra weight comes

There are times in your life when you must guard carefully against the perilous probability of weight gain. Like many others, you may allow a few too many extra pounds to accumulate after achieving adulthood—probably because of reduced physical activity with no change in food intake. Don't let those added pounds go unnoticed.

As you grow older, your body requires fewer calories to fuel basic processes. Unless food intake is gradually reduced or physical activity increased, extra pounds will surely sneak up.

Women tend to gain weight at menopause and after the birth of children, especially if the first child comes when the woman is in her thirties.

Excess weight carried over from childhood can be a lifelong problem requiring constant vigilance. Sometimes emotional or psychological problems related to being overweight need medical attention.

Fallacies about reducing

Misconceptions about reducing explain the appeal of many get-slim-quick schemes which seem to promise that you can lose those excess pounds with no effort at all.

Novel diets of supposedly superior slimming power keep springing up and fading away. Sometimes it is implied that the calories of certain foods or beverages are ignored by the body and that these foods can be eaten in any quantities. But calories always count, whatever their source. The only calories that don't count are those you don't swallow.

Sometimes, incredible virtues are attributed to exotic foods, or to one or two foods at the expense of others, although common wholesome foods in variety are the best and safest foundation for reducing diets.

Food Exchanges provide a seemingly endless variety of nutritious foods that can be the basis of a well-balanced reducing diet. No question about it: Only the magic of a balanced reducing diet can result in years of eating and staying slim and healthy. The Food Exchange system provides good eating habits that help keep off unwanted pounds.

Massage, by hand or with vibrators, has valuable uses, but not for reducing. Fat won't melt away or rub off through massage. Local fat deposits can't be reduced by rollers or by shaking, shimmying gadgets. If so-called "spot reducing" techniques seem to get results, it's because the subject has been made to eat less, get more exercise, or both. Passive exercise (the kind in which all the effort is provided by another person or by a motor-driven machine) is useless for shedding fat or increasing muscle strength. This exercise system, however, may make you feel good.

Water is a part of your total body weight. Sweating from strenuous exercise, a hot bath, or baking in a steam cabinet can get rid of a pound or two in a hurry. But what you lose is merely water which is promptly replaced when you drink. Body fat can't be steamed off effectively.

"Reducing pills" prescribed by doctors are potent drugs, available only by prescription. Most common pills act on centers of the brain to depress appetite. This may make a low-calorie diet more satisfying during the first few weeks when the reducer is adjusting to the different diet and learning better eating habits.

Another drug prescribed by physicians is thyroid substance, which makes body fires burn more brightly. A few people who produce too little thyroid hormone may be sluggish and overweight and are prescribed thyroid substance. However, if a person's thyroid production is normal (tests by your doctor are necessary to determine this), additional thyroid supplements can be hazardous to your health.

The place of drugs in weight reduction is simple. If your doctor prescribes them, take them. If he doesn't prescribe them for you, then leave them alone and avoid potential problems.

chapter 3

calorie calculations

A pound of fat body tissue contains about 3,500 calories, about the same number as a pound of butter.

So the arithmetic of reducing is simple. Subtract 3,500 calories and you shed a pound of fat. Subtract 7,000 calories and you shed two pounds.

Of course, this takes a bit of doing. But it's heartening to know that it needn't, or shouldn't, be done all at once. You can set your own reducing speed, within limits.

Take in 1,000 fewer calories a day than you burn up and you should lose about two pounds in a week—about the maximum rate of fat loss that most doctors think

desirable without close medical supervision. Or you can subtract only 500 calories a day, and lose about a pound a week.

Actual weight loss on a reducing diet may be greater or less than you expect and may have its ups and downs. There are modifying factors such as fluid retention (see page 13). But the difference between caloric intake (food) and output (energy expenditure) basically determines your reducing speed. Remember, when your caloric intake exceeds your caloric output, weight is gained, and when your caloric output exceeds your caloric intake, weight is lost.

Figuring your daily calorie needs

How many calories a day do you need to maintain your normal weight, neither gaining nor losing?

Most moderately active people require about 15 calories per pound of desirable weight (see page 6). Multiply your desirable or ideal weight by 15 to calculate the number of calories you need to maintain that weight. Thus, if you wish to maintain your weight at 100 pounds, you can eat foods containing no more than 1,500 calories.

There are individual differences of size and shape, and variations in calorie needs, but for practical purposes, the figure of 15 calories per pound gives a yardstick of desirable calorie intake by men and women who aren't running marathons or playing basketball all day long. Be careful not to confuse active and busy. A busy person who remains seated all day is not necessarily an active person.

Remember that these calories are *maintenance* calories. To shed fat, you'll have to consume fewer calories than those needed to maintain your ideal weight. Figure it this way if you're a moderately active person, weighing 100 pounds:

Maintenance calories	1500
Subtract calories furnished by reducing diet	−1000
Daily calorie deficit	500

The 100-pound body requires and burns 1,500 calories daily: 1,000 calories are furnished by the reducing diet and the remaining 500 calories come from fat stored in the body. That's what makes the fat go away—*withdrawals* from the fat bank.

To calculate the approximate reducing speed, divide the daily calorie deficit into 3,500 calories per pound of fat body tissue. This equals the number of days it takes to lose a pound of fat body tissue. For the person in our example it would be figured as follows:

$$3,500 \div 500 = 7 \text{ days}$$

Actual weight loss usually is greater because some water is lost with the fat.

Choose one of the Food Exchange reducing plans of 1,000, 1,200, or 1,500 calories (page 36) and estimate your reducing speed as explained above. You can't be exact to the last ounce or even half pound, but you can come close enough. Ultimately, your body is the most infallible calorie counter of all and will tell you how you're doing.

More exercise, less fat

Would you like to lose fat just as fast on a 1,500-calorie reducing diet as on a 1,000-calorie reducing diet?

It could be done by increasing your physical activity 500 calories worth. Like walking at a moderate clip for two and one-half hours.

That may be more exercise than you care for. An easier route to slimness may be the reduction of food intake. But you may not be able to win a lifetime victory over weight unless you combine an increase in physical activity with reduction of calorie intake. Whichever route you select, your daily calorie intake must be less than the energy you expend in order to lose weight.

Fat tends to accumulate after age 25 because body metabolism and physical activity tend to dwindle while food intake remains the same. Pounds pile up slowly even without increased food intake.

It's surprising how many calories can be burned by a small daily increase in exercise. A moderate 20-minute walk burns only 70 calories. But keep it up every day for seven weeks and you subtract 3,500 calories—the equivalent of a pound of fat.

Diet and exercise "mystery" solved

Differences in physical activity explain some of the supposed "mysteries" of excess weight. For instance, an obese woman may say: "I eat less than my slim friends but still gain weight. It must be my glands." It is possible that she does gain weight while eating less than others who do not gain. But glands rarely have much to do with it.

One study of overly fat women showed that they ate less than women of normal weight. But they also spent about two-thirds less time in activities involving significant amounts of exercise. Another study of overweight adolescent girls showed that they spent much less energy during exercise periods than their slim counterparts. In fact, they coasted a lot.

Overweight women in these studies got fat although they weren't enormous eaters. They simply took in more calories than they burned. There was no mystery about it. The amount of food they consumed was considerably more than that required to maintain their weight. Don't be fooled into thinking that you gained weight while eating like a bird.

Burning calories by exercising

If giving up 500 or 1,000 calories a day sounds like an impossible task for you, consider stepping up your physical activity. Keeping fit through regular exercise burns calories and firms flabby muscles as well. Have no fear of developing large unattractive bulges from calisthenics and other physical activities. Instead, your appearance will improve as newly toned muscles provide better support for your body. And, your exercise program should not completely drain you of all energy. Rather, you should feel full of new-found vitality and charged with energy you never thought you had.

Here are estimates by the American Medical Association of the number of calories burned per hour performing several kinds of activities:

activity	calories/hour
lying down, sitting	70-100
office work, domestic chores, driving	120-180
walking and bicycling (moderate speed)	200-220
golf, heavy housework, bowling, walking (briskly)	250-300
volleyball, skating, jogging, dancing, tennis, swimming	350-450
competitive sports such as running, rowing, swimming	600+

Take care when calculating the calorie-cost of your activities. Calories expended during exercise vary with the intensity of performance. Very few people swim for an hour at top speed. Some people burn more calories while sitting than others. The lean ones will fuss and twitch, change position, gnash their teeth, or grip a pencil tightly. More placid and more upholstered people just sit and relax. And certain individuals will perform a task more efficiently than others, burning fewer calories. The number of calories used per hour is also affected by an individual's size, age, sex, and other factors. These differences aside, one factor remains: Exercise affects your rate of weight loss.

To demonstrate how a little added exercise can help you stay slim, let's take a fairly measurable form of exercise—walking at 3.5 miles per hour —and figure approximately how long it takes to burn up calories from several familiar foods:

food	Time required to burn food walking at 3.5 m.p.h.
large apple	20 minutes
bacon (2 slices)	18 minutes
glass of beer	22 minutes
doughnut	30 minutes
hard-cooked egg	15 minutes
hamburger	70 minutes
apple pie (1/6)	75 minutes
ice cream soda	50 minutes
soft drink	20 minutes

What kind of exercise?

Regular exercise is far better than occasional bursts of strenuous activity. Things we enjoy doing are best because things we like are habit-forming, and exercise should become a habit that we don't have to nudge ourselves into grudgingly because it's "good for us." That is why it's important that you develop an exercise program tailored to your daily lifestyle. Let exercising become a lifelong fitness program. Walking, swimming, jogging, dancing, mowing the lawn, spading the garden—you name it and it's fine as long as you stop short of fatigue.

If you're really serious about a regular exercise program, be sure to include a regimen of exercise for flexibility (stretching), circulation (walking, running, jumping rope, bicycling, etc.), and strength (squats, push-ups, chin-ups, sit-ups, etc.). Engage in physical activity whenever the opportunity arises (use stairs instead of the elevator, or park your car farther away from where you work) and be ready for lots of supplementary physical recreation—volleyball, softball, bowling, ice-skating, basketball—whatever activity you prefer. The intensity of any activity will affect its weight-loss value.

Select a regular time for your exercise program, and make it part of your daily routine. It's best to exercise three or four hours after a meal. Don't quit at the first drop of perspiration, but you needn't push yourself to the point of discomfort, either. Start your program slowly with a few exercises and add others each day as your fitness improves. Don't get discouraged, because improvement takes time.

chapter 4

basics of reducing

A low-calorie diet does not provide the dieter with as many calories as the body burns in its activities. To make up this deficit, calories must be subtracted from fat body tissue. Otherwise, a low-calorie diet could "steal" from vital organs, muscles, and

tissues. A reducing diet should provide all the essentials except calories. A reducing diet based on Food Exchanges will provide adequate nutrients for most people. A variety of foods will help ensure that your diet is nutritionally adequate.

Elements of good nutrition

Protein is of primary importance to all living things. It is essential for growth and repair of tissue and for providing the spark that speeds chemical activities of body cells. The foods which furnish top quality proteins are usually of animal origin, although vegetable protein sources make a significant nutritional contribution.

Fats and oils (liquid fats) are essential in the diet. They provide "staying power" to meals and weight for weight contain more than twice as many calories

as carbohydrates or proteins. This, unfortunately, makes them deceptive; they can load a menu with more calories than reducers expect or want. Much of the fat we eat is "invisible," in meats, dairy products, and eggs, or is added during the preparation of food.

Carbohydrate foods (starches and sugars) furnish much of the energy for body activities. They free protein for other uses, help the body burn fat efficiently, and are inexpensive and important carriers of vitamins and minerals. Most of our carbohydrates come from vegetables, cereals, and fruits. Dairy products furnish some carbohydrates, meats provide virtually none.

What to expect when reducing

Diets can be standardized, but people can't. Individual factors such as amount of exercise or fluid retention can affect the apparent speed of reducing. It is quite possible to lose *fat* although for a time the scales may show little or no *weight* loss.

Allowing for individual variation, experienced physicians generally agree on some broad generalizations about reducing:

The greatest weight loss for most people on a reducing diet usually occurs during the first week, and the major weight loss usually occurs during the first month.

Weight loss may hit a plateau and level off at the end of four to six weeks. Don't be discouraged. It's probably a good sign that the body is adapting to a lower calorie intake, which is needed to maintain your weight loss. Don't fall off the reducing wagon; pounds will come off, but at a slower rate.

Fluid retention and weight loss

If your weight loss is less one day than another, don't be surprised. Expect it. Few reducers show consistent, unvarying weight loss from week to week. The scales may show considerable fluctuation, up today, down tomorrow. Often this reflects changes in salt and fluid balances of the body. Every pint of retained fluid equals one pound of weight (not fat). This can "hide" fat loss that has occurred. Generally, fluid fluctuations are greatest in the first stages of reducing, after which the body "settles down" and the scales more truthfully reflect actual fat loss.

Restriction of salt in the diet tends to give a more even rate of weight reduction. Common salt holds a certain amount of water in the body and tends to stimulate eating by making things taste better. It also provokes thirst and fluid intake. So instead of reaching for the salt shaker when you cook, consider other excellent flavor enhancers such as spices and herbs. They will bolster the taste of many of your favorite foods.

Retained fluids come not only from water, but also from other beverages and, in fact, from food. When the body breaks food into its various components, one of the by-products is water.

In summary, it's a good idea to go easy on the salt shaker and to avoid highly salted foods—such as potato chips—when reducing.

For that filled-up feeling

A well-balanced reducing diet is never a starvation diet for anyone with fat to lose. The so-called hunger pangs of reducing are usually not caused by hunger, but by appetite, quite a different matter.

If you're serious about shedding pounds, take careful account of your eating habits—the where, the way, the why, the what, and of course, how much. Once you see your eating pattern, you can pinpoint your problem areas. Do you skip meals, then gorge later to compensate? Do you snack on high-calorie foods? Does your diet include too much sugar? Fat? Do you eat to be sociable, even if you're not hungry? When you're thirsty do you reach for a soft drink rather than water?

Eating is a highly individual matter so you may find that your problem is none of the above. But there is one unalterable fact that must be faced by anyone who wants to lose weight: Losing pounds requires burning up more calories than you consume. Here are several tricks that can help you stretch a low-calorie diet into a lot of eating satisfaction:

Fragment your meals. You can stretch your daily food allowance into four, five, or six small meals to keep your stomach satisfyingly busy.

Take your time. Savor each morsel. Take small bits. Play the gourmet, connoisseur of flavors. This ploy can slow the eating momentum which could propel you into consuming more than you really want. It takes a little time for food you have eaten to tell you that you are filled up.

Don't eat when you're not hungry. Silly advice? Well, have you ever eaten bridge-game tidbits for the same reason that men climb mountains: "Because they're there"? Or taken a piece of cake to please a hostess? Or nibbled to pass the time?

Limit the areas where you eat. Eat all your meals and snacks in the kitchen or dining room; consider all other rooms out of bounds. Concentrate on eating. Sometimes you just don't realize how much you're eating when you're reading or watching television at the same time.

Don't keep your goal a secret. The support of your family and friends can strengthen your resolve. Make your goals realistic or you may be disappointed.

Use foods with Free Exchange ratings. Make meals more appetizing with herbs, spices, and other "free" condiments (see page 30).

Lettuce, radishes, escarole, or endive, low-calorie flavored gelatin, and low-calorie carbonated beverages are just right for snacks. Coffee and tea are "free" too.

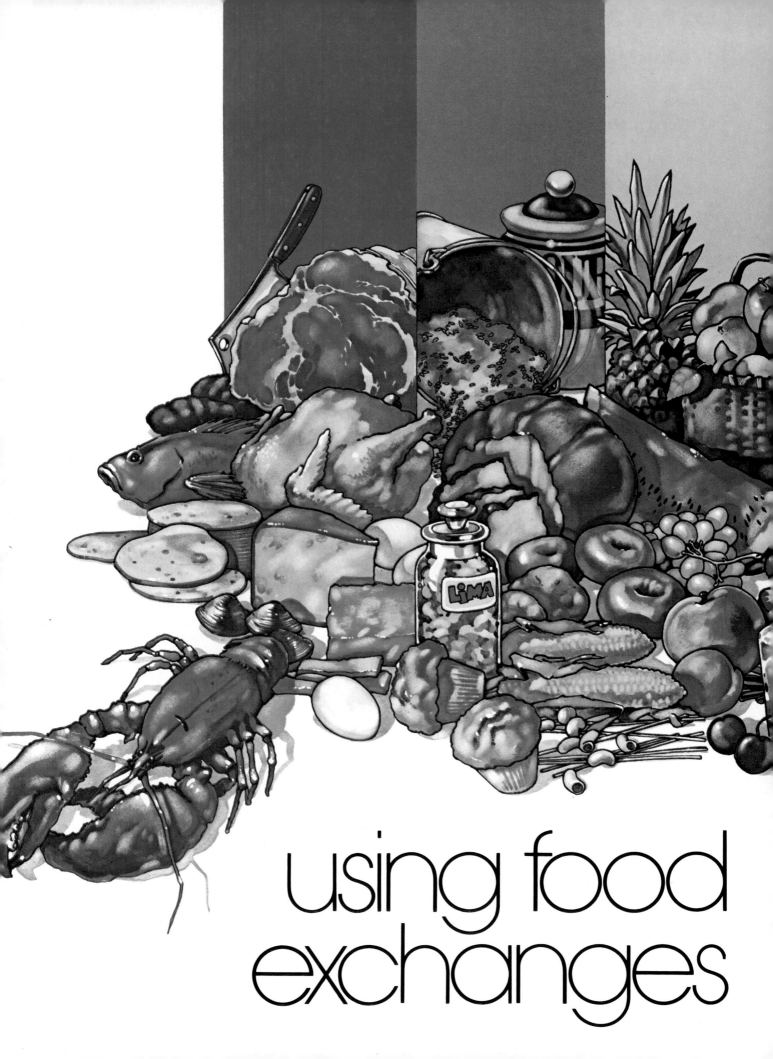

using food
exchanges

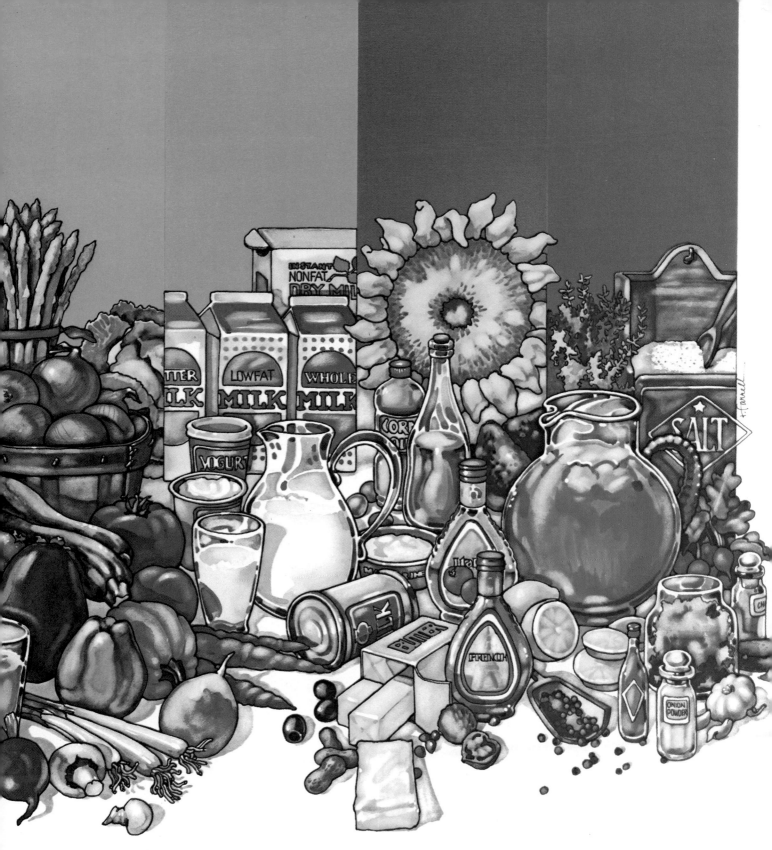

Let Food Exchanges count calories for you as you choose foods from the seven groups displayed on these pages. Make your mealtime selections from the color-coded Exchanges—Meat, Bread, Fruit, Vegetable, Milk, Fat, and Free—based on the Daily Meal Plan of your choice (page 36). Once you master the system, using it will become second nature. You can shed unwanted pounds and keep them off for good.

using food exchanges

Don't let the term Food Exchange intimidate you. Although it sounds very technical, it's really a simple method used for many years by dietitians to balance diets carefully.

There's nothing intimidating about the Food Exchanges in this book. Each Food Exchange is merely a measurement of calorie and nutrient values. Foods are divided into seven Exchange groups—Meat, Bread, Fruit, Vegetable, Milk, Fat, and a group of Free foods. The foods in each Exchange group contain similar amounts of proteins, fats, carbohydrates, and calories.

A Bread Exchange isn't necessarily bread. It can be a tortilla, cereal, or peas. Any differences in nutrients and calories are adjusted by the serving size. Because one slice of white bread furnishes the same amount of proteins, carbohydrates, and calories as one tortilla, one-half cup of peas, or one cup of puffed cereal, all count as one Bread Exchange. Thus, they can be interchanged on a menu. That is why the seven food groups are called Food "Exchanges." And, by using them in your daily eating pattern, a varied diet is assured. It's easier to stay on a diet that has variety.

Understanding the Food Exchange Lists

Food Exchanges can simplify reducing for you by counting calories, assuring a well-balanced diet, permitting you to choose the foods you like best within a food group, and providing menus easily adapted for all members of the family.

Look at the Food Exchange Lists on pages 26-30. The foods included are bulwarks of the everyday American diet. Each list has a color symbol for recognition at a glance.

- ● Lean Meat Exchange
- ● Bread Exchange
- ○ Fruit Exchange
- ● Vegetable Exchange
- ● Milk Exchange
- ● Fat Exchange
- ● Free Exchange

The size of each serving is specified. Exchange units are usually expressed as ounces or as standard measuring cups and spoons. It is important that you be able to estimate and visualize these measures accurately. At first you may want to measure servings using standard measuring cups and spoons. But after a while, you'll be able to recognize quantities such as one-half cup of peas or one cup of puffed cereal. A small dietary scale may be useful for weighing meat.

Take a look at the Meat Exchange List on pages 26-27. You'll find it divided into three subcategories according to fat content. The three subcategories are Lean Meat, Medium-Fat Meat, and High-Fat Meat. These may be easier to think of as fat, fatter, and fattest. The Lean Meat Exchange provides seven grams of protein, three grams of fat, and 55 calories per serving. The Medium-Fat Meat Exchange provides seven grams of protein and five and one-half grams of fat. It contains 75 calories per serving because of its higher fat content. You must charge yourself an extra one-half Fat Exchange above and beyond the Lean Meat Exchange for each serving of Medium-Fat Meat. Each serving of High-Fat Meat provides seven grams of protein, eight grams of fat, and 100 calories. It costs one additional Fat Exchange.

But why all the calculations and talk about calories? There's no need for you to compute or worry about calories. When necessary, simply account for the appropriate number of Fat Exchanges per serving of Medium- or High-Fat Meat. You'll find all the meal plans and recipes in this book are based on the Lean Meat Exchange plus a specified number of Fat Exchanges when Medium- or High-Fat Meats are used.

As you might expect, the Bread Exchange List on page 28 contains bread, cereals, and crackers. But it also lists dried beans and starchy vegetables such as corn, peas, and potatoes. At first glance, you may think the potatoes are out of place. Not so. One small potato delivers about the same cargo of proteins, carbohydrates, and calories as does one slice of bread. Also contained in the Bread Exchange List are various prepared foods for which one or two additional Fat Exchanges must be deducted when figuring Food Exchanges.

No complicating factors are found in the Fruit Exchange List on page 29, because all fruits are fat-free. One fruit, cranberries, can be eaten to your heart's content as long as no sugar is added.

Most vegetables can be found in the Vegetable Exchange List on page 29. As mentioned, dried beans and starchy vegetables are found in the Bread Exchange List. Some raw vegetables (chicory, chinese cabbage, endive, escarole, lettuce, parsley, radishes, and watercress) can be eaten in any amount and merit a coveted Free Exchange rating.

The Milk Exchange List on page 29 is based on nonfat milk. Thus, if you choose an item from this list *not* made from nonfat or skim milk, you must account for the equivalent Fat Exchanges.

Fat Exchanges, found on page 30, include nuts, olives, and avocados, in addition to the more common fats and oils. The Fat Exchange List probably tells you more than you ever wanted to know about saturated and unsaturated fats.

In the Free Exchange List on page 30, you'll find flavor bonuses such as salt, pepper, herbs, and spices. A variety of other foods and beverages are offered to please your palate and fill you up without adding significant calories.

Not at all hard to understand, is it? Now you're ready to put the Food Exchanges to work.

Easy meal planning

The Daily Meal Plans (page 36) give you a choice of three "reducing speeds" — 1,000, 1,200, or 1,500 calories a day. Choose a meal plan with a daily calorie deficit that lets you reduce no more than two pounds a week (pages 9-11). From now on, think no more about counting calories.

Just select the foods you like from the respective Food Exchange Lists specified for each meal. For example, on the 1,000-calorie diet you are allowed one Fruit Exchange for breakfast. The Fruit Exchange List gives you many choices—one-half small banana, one fig if you feel exotic, or one-half cup unsweetened applesauce if you don't. Remember to read the Food Exchange Lists carefully. Serving sizes differ within a Food Exchange group and may be somewhat different from the serving sizes you are accustomed to eating.

Go over the other specified Food Exchanges for breakfast, lunch, and dinner on page 36, and make your selections from the Food Exchange Lists on pages 26-30. Choose any food you desire, as long as it fits into a Daily Meal Plan that helps you lose about two pounds in a week. One warning: If you exceed the Exchange allotments of your Daily Meal Plan, your reducing progress will be slow.

On the 1,000-calorie daily diet, you are allowed one Lean Meat Exchange at breakfast, two Lean Meat Exchanges at lunch, and two Lean Meat Exchanges at dinner. As an example, let's make appropriate meat selections for each of the three meals and incorporate them in the 1,000-calorie Daily Meal Plan.

A typical Meat Exchange selection at breakfast might be a poached egg. But you won't find eggs on the Lean Meat Exchange. They're on the Medium-Fat Exchange. In this case, just deduct one-half Fat Exchange in addition to one Lean Meat Exchange from the breakfast meal plan.

At lunch, when two Lean Meat Exchanges are allotted, cottage cheese would be a logical choice. One Lean Meat Exchange is equivalent to one-fourth cup cottage cheese (2% butterfat), so two Exchanges would allow one-half cup cottage cheese (2% butterfat) at lunchtime.

At dinnertime, you could choose frankfurters as your Meat Exchanges, but only if you deduct one Fat Exchange in addition to one Lean Meat Exchange per frankfurter (because frankfurters are found on the High-Fat Meat Exchange List). So in order to fit two frankfurters into the dinner meal plan for the 1,000-calorie diet, you would have to subtract two Fat Exchanges in addition to two Lean Meat Exchanges. That takes care of the dinnertime allotment of both Meat and Fat Exchanges.

Breakfast and dinner meal plans on page 36 allow only one-half of a Milk Exchange at each meal. In this case, choose any item from the Milk Exchange List, but cut the quantity in half. For example, for one-half of a Milk Exchange, you may have one-half cup of skim milk instead of the one cup for a full Exchange.

Your selection of foods will add up automatically in round numbers to the number of calories in the Daily Meal Plan you choose. The number of Food Exchanges specified in your Daily Meal Plan takes care of the arithmetic for you. What a relief to make easy choices of your favorite foods instead of counting calories! Together, the Food Exchange List and the Daily Meal Plans will add variety and spice to all your meals.

Helpful meal planning hints

The Daily Meal Plans show the conventional three meals a day. But no law requires three. You can divide your allotted Food Exchanges for the day into half a dozen small meals or three meals plus a coffee break or bedtime snack. In fact, spreading your supply of Food Exchanges over the entire day may help you to reduce hunger pangs between meals.

If you carry a lunch, you might want to borrow a breakfast or dinner bread allowance in order to enjoy a lunchbox sandwich. Or you may be content with the Bread Exchanges the way they are.

Remember, you can substitute one food for another in the same Food Exchange List, but you can't substitute foods of one Exchange List for foods of a different Exchange. You can't swap grapefruit juice for cottage cheese without risk of upsetting dietary balance or calorie contribution. Let the color code of the Food Exchange Lists be your guide. Substitute only those foods with the same color code. The Bread and Fruit Exchanges are the exceptions. Refer to pages 21 and 22 to find out how to substitute fruit for bread or vice-versa.

"Mixed" foods, such as stews or casseroles, combine foods from different Exchange Lists. Their composition can be calculated closely enough by dissecting them to determine the Meat, Bread, Fruit, Vegetable, Milk, Fat, or Free Exchanges that compose them. This was the procedure used to calculate the recipes on pages 50-81. This dissection doesn't always give you enough calories or nutrients to equal one whole Food Exchange. As a result, one-half and sometimes even one-fourth Food Exchanges are used. Look for the following color symbols:

● 1 Milk Exchange

◖ ½ Milk Exchange

◤ ¼ Milk Exchange

Round out fractional Exchanges with partial servings of that particular Exchange.

The Menu Planning Steps and sample menus (pages 37-49) are a good place to begin your menu planning. We've devised several menus for the 1,000-, 1,200-, and 1,500-calorie Daily Meal Plans. You'll find them helpful for getting started.

Built-in daily variety

Endless variety is built into the Daily Meal Plans. Take full advantage of it when making your Food Exchange selections. Variety comes close to being a magic word in nutrition. Too much of one type of food or too little of another makes a diet lopsided. A *balance* of a variety of foods is the key to proper nutrition. The foods in each Exchange group make a specific nutritional contribution. No single Food Exchange group can supply all the nutrients needed for a well-balanced diet. It takes foods from all of the Exchange groups to supply your nutritional needs for good health.

The Daily Meal Plans furnish a fine balance of essential nutrients in the most convenient way. You can substitute foods that you happen to have on hand, foods that are in season and inexpensive when plentiful, or those you just happen to like best. If there's no bread in the cupboard, but there is a small leftover boiled potato in the refrigerator, it's nice to know that you can substitute the potato for the bread. Making such choices provides variety in a mixed diet. The Food Exchange Lists are indeed good mixers.

Add to the Food Exchange Lists the recipes starting on page 50 and your mealtime choices grow. Tastefully seasoned, these imaginative recipes are based on Food Exchanges for easy incorporation into the Daily Meal Plans. These recipes are easy and almost as sumptuous as any calorie-laden food you've ever tasted. You can indulge yourself with these dishes as long as you account for the appropriate number of Food Exchanges from your Daily Meal Plan. Non-dieting families and friends will also enjoy the reducing recipes.

Also found on the following pages are Exchange Lists for Packaged Foods (pages 31-35). Designed to unravel the mysteries of packaged foods, these lists translate technical nutrition information into the easy-to-use Exchanges. Now you can eliminate the guesswork and use convenience foods confidently—even if you're dieting.

Because many meals are eaten outside the home, we've included simple, common sense suggestions on dining out. They start on page 86. You also will find a clip-out guide to many popular American chain restaurants on page 89. It shows Exchange ratings for several common menu items.

The choices are yours. Select foods to fit your Daily Meal Plan from the variety of foods found on the Exchange Lists, the Exchange Lists for Packaged Foods, the clip-out Restaurant Exchanges, or the recipes found in this book. Then, enjoy a different menu each day.

Food Exchanges to hold your weight loss

The Daily Meal Plans are deficient only in calories (that's why they make excess fat disappear). After you have reduced to your ideal weight using the Daily Meal Plans, you will need more calories—but not a great number more—to maintain your weight without putting a load of fat back on your frame.

With your eating habits geared to weight reduction, it will be easy to increase your caloric intake to maintenance levels (page 94). You can use the Daily Meal Plans as the foundation of a balanced diet. For example, while keeping the same balance of good nutrition, you can increase the calories by adding a few extra servings from the Food Exchanges. You will recognize the values of the different Food Exchanges almost instinctively by the time you reach the happy stage when you need more calories to keep from wasting away to a shadow.

Food Exchanges can help ensure a lifetime of good balanced eating. Give them a try. Food is one of life's basic necessities, and eating one of its greatest pleasures.

POINTS TO REMEMBER

One Food Exchange: A measurement of calorie and nutrient values. Foods within the same Exchange can be interchanged; they contain similar amounts of nutrients and calories in each specified serving.

Food Exchange Lists: Seven lists of foods. Foods in each list have similar amounts of protein, fat, carbohydrate, and calories. Caloric values within an Exchange group are adjusted by serving size.

Daily Meal Plans: A daily guide of reducing menus which counts the calories for you (page 36).

meat exchange

The Meat Exchanges (pages 26-27) are the protein keystones of your meals. For good reason, the meat course is the pièce de résistance. Meat Exchanges aren't limited to poultry, meat, and fish. They include a variety of top-notch protein foods.

All the foods found in the Meat Exchange List provide generous amounts of protein, the nutrient responsible for tissue building and repair. Many members of the Meat Exchange family are good sources of the B vitamins and minerals such as iron, zinc, and phosphorous. Foods in the Meat Exchange List contain similar amounts of all nutrients except fat. The Medium- and High-Fat Meat Exchanges contain more fat than the Lean Meat Exchange. Foods from the Medium-Fat Meat Exchange cost one-half additional Fat Exchange (except peanut butter, which costs two and one-half additional Fat Exchanges), while foods from the High-Fat Meat Exchange cost one additional Fat Exchange per serving.

Most foods in the Lean Meat Exchange are low in cholesterol and saturated fat. Peanut butter (a Medium-Fat Meat Exchange) contains no cholesterol and is also low in saturated fat. Cholesterol is produced by the body or supplied by foods of animal origin. It is a constituent of plaque, a substance which can settle within the walls of blood vessels and has been implicated in various forms of heart disease. Saturated fats also come from animal sources. A large proportion of saturated fats in the diet may increase the level of cholesterol in the blood. Medical experts recommend that heavy consumption of cholesterol and saturated fat be avoided.

Most Exchanges are based on one-ounce servings of *cooked* meat. A three-ounce serving of cooked meat is about equal to four ounces of raw meat. Trim all fat from meat. If meat is fried, count the fat used to fry it as a Fat Exchange. To brown meat, use a pan with a non-stick surface or use a small amount of diet imitation margarine.

Don't forget about seafood. One ounce of any fresh, frozen, or canned seafood is equivalent to one Lean Meat Exchange. Be sure to drain all canned seafood well and use water-pack when possible. In practical measures, one-fourth cup of canned salmon, tuna, or mackerel is equivalent to one Lean Meat Exchange. That's also true for crab and lobster in any form. Five scallops, shrimp, oysters, or clams, or three *drained* sardines equal one Lean Meat Exchange.

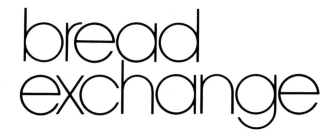

bread exchange

The Bread Exchange (page 28) is a versatile group. This all-around category includes cereals, crackers, dried beans, starchy vegetables, bread, and prepared foods. Bread Exchanges all contain similar amounts of nutrients.

The Bread Exchanges are your daily packets of energy. Bread Exchanges, together with Vegetable and Fruit Exchanges, furnish carbohydrates, which are primary fuels for moving muscles and keeping body fires burning. Carbohydrates "spare" protein for other valuable functions and help the body burn fat efficiently. As you can see, carbohydrates are an important part of the diet.

Bread Exchanges give us important B vitamins and minerals necessary for normal body functions. Whole-grain and enriched breads and cereals, as well as dried beans and peas, are good sources of iron (a mineral) and are among the better sources of thiamin (a B vitamin). Germ and bran products are also important sources of iron and thiamin. Potatoes contribute a little vitamin C to the diet while sweet potatoes contribute a good deal of vitamin A. Potassium and folacin are also provided by some foods in the Bread Exchange.

Fiber, an important constituent of today's diet, is provided by whole-grain, bran, and germ products. Dried beans and peas also are good sources of fiber. Fiber or roughage in the diet aids in normal elimination of body wastes. Scientists believe other possible

health benefits are associated with fiber. The protein content of the Bread Exchanges (except dried peas and beans) is not high when compared with the protein of the Meat and Milk Exchange Lists, but it is nevertheless important. It constitutes a major source of protein for many people of the world.

Except for the prepared Bread Exchanges, there is almost no fat in the Bread Exchange group.

Sugars and syrups are concentrated forms of carbohydrate. They are less desirable for reducers than foods from the Bread, Fruit, and Vegetable Exchanges which provide vital vitamins and minerals in addition to the carbohydrate and calories they furnish.

You'll find the Bread Exchanges are easy to fit into your Daily Meal Plan. At breakfast, you can combine cereals with milk and fruit. Add non-caloric sweetener if you desire. At lunch, serve an assortment of crackers to accompany soups and salads. Serve graham crackers with a glass of milk for a snack. And don't forget the prepared foods—biscuits, muffins, pancakes, waffles, French-fried potatoes, and potato chips. But remember they'll cost you one or two extra Fat Exchanges.

The number of Bread Exchanges on the Daily Meal Plans may not be enough for bread lovers. If that's the case, you may wish to substitute one Bread Exchange for one and one-half Fruit Exchanges on any of the Daily Meal Plans.

fruit exchange

Fruit Exchanges (page 29) are full of flavor and nutrition. Sweet by nature, they don't need any added sweetening, certainly not if you're dieting. You can savor the natural goodness of fruit any time of the day. You'll find fruit a refreshing addition to meals and satisfying as a snack.

Just about all the calories in fruits come from the sugars and other carbohydrates which supply energy for body activities. Fruits are valuable for their vitamins, minerals, and fiber. Fruits are rich sources of vitamin C, which is needed in relatively large quantities compared to other vitamins. Vitamin C is particularly abundant in citrus fruits and juices. Many fruits are also valuable for their vitamin A. The better sources of vitamin A among the fruits are fresh or dried apricots, mangoes, cantaloupe, nectarines, yellow peaches, and persimmons. Fruits are well-known as rich sources of potassium, an essential mineral. Other important vitamins and minerals are also present in fruit.

Exchanges for fruits are based on fresh fruit unless specified. Canned, frozen, or dried fruit can be substituted as long as no sugar is added. When substituting canned fruit for fresh fruit, use either *unsweetened* fruit (water-pack) or *artificially sweetened* fruit (dietetic-pack). You'll be adding unwanted calories if you use juice or syrup-pack fruit. Read labels carefully.

Fruits are unbeatable for flavor and eyecatching color. They're a tasty addition to meals and snacks.

Fruits are a healthy way to start each day, diet or no diet. But to avoid that everyday orange juice routine, eat a variety of fruits with berries, grapefruit, and melon at the top of the list. Enjoy plumped raisins or bananas on your cereal. Or,

indulge yourself with something a little more exotic —perhaps a tropical fruit cup consisting of papaya, pineapple, and mango.

At lunchtime, fruit salads are limited only by your imagination. Try fruit molded in your favorite flavor of low-calorie gelatin, or team it up with cottage cheese or yogurt. Sample pears stuffed with cream cheese and served on a bed of lettuce. And to add a new twist to your chicken salad, serve it atop pineapple rings. Try adding a fruit accent to a tossed green salad. Mandarin orange slices and fresh torn spinach are a good combination.

There's no need to fall off the dieting wagon when it comes to dessert. You'll find fruit can be delightfully sweet and every bit as enticing as any calorie-rich dessert you've ever eaten. For many luscious fruit desserts, see recipes beginning on page 76.

If you're really a fruit lover, the three Fruit Exchanges allowed on the Daily Meal Plan may not be enough. If that's the case, substitute one and one-half Fruit Exchanges for one Bread Exchange on the Daily Meal Plan.

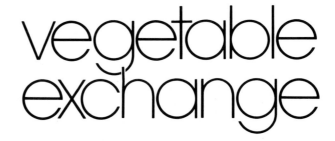

vegetable exchange

Not only are Vegetable Exchanges (page 29) great to taste, but they also supply valuable vitamins and minerals. The generous use of an assortment of nutritious vegetables in your diet contributes to sound health and vitality. Enjoy them cooked or raw.

Among the leading sources of vitamin A in the diet are the dark green and deep yellow members of the Vegetable Exchange. In addition, many of the vegetables of this group are notable sources of vitamin C, with asparagus, broccoli, brussels sprouts, beet greens, cabbage, cauliflower, collards, kale, dandelion, mustard and turnip greens, spinach, rutabagas, tomatoes, and turnips leading the way. Fiber, which helps promote regularity, is present in vegetables. Vegetables are loaded with other important vitamins and minerals, too.

Whether you serve them cooked or raw, wash all vegetables even though they may look clean. If fat is added in preparation, omit the equivalent number of Fat Exchanges. Add zest without adding Exchanges to vegetables by cooking with herbs and spices. Start with about one-fourth teaspoon of the desired herb or spice per four servings. Cook vegetables in nonfat beef or chicken broth for a free flavor bonus.

Vegetable salads serve the dieter in good stead, but be adventuresome! Start with a variety of greens (endive, escarole, bibb or Boston lettuce—they're all free), add a few of your favorite raw vegetables, and dress with low-calorie dressing.

Toss it together and presto—a self-styled salad. When you need a change from tossed green salads, capture your favorite vegetable in a molded vegetable salad. Use unflavored or low-calorie gelatin (lemon or lime flavors supply just the right pizzazz).

Complement spinach, broccoli, brussels sprouts, asparagus, or green beans with vinegar or a lemon wedge. Top with cheese or croutons, but deduct the appropriate Exchanges. When you want to break away from the commonplace, skewer an assortment of vegetable tidbits, brush with low-calorie dressing, and broil or grill till they're sizzling. If you prefer cold vegetables, marinate with low-calorie salad dressing overnight in the refrigerator, drain, and serve atop ice-cold lettuce.

Treat yourself to a glass of tomato juice or vegetable juice cocktail as an appetizer or snack. Dash in a squirt of lemon juice, worcestershire sauce, or bottled hot pepper sauce. Sprinkle lightly with seasoned salt, onion salt, or celery salt for a change of pace. A radish rose tops it off with added flair without adding any Food Exchanges (other than a Free one).

Speaking of snacktime, don't forget vegetable relishes. Devour radishes to your heart's content, but be sure to measure amounts of other vegetables such as celery, carrots, cucumbers, or cauliflower. One-half cup equals one Vegetable Exchange.

milk exchange

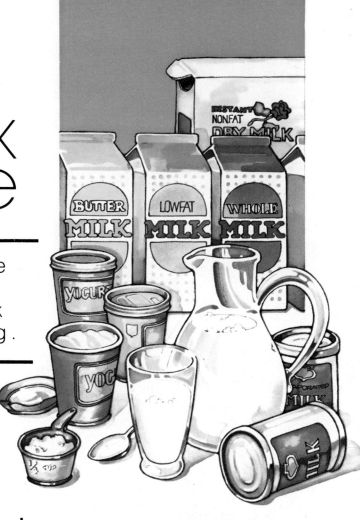

The Milk Exchanges (page 29) are not for drinking only. Excellent sources of nutrients, milk and milk products are often used for cooking .

Milk is the leading source of dietary calcium. It supplies protein of top quality and contains vitamins A and D, B vitamins, phosphorus, and magnesium.

The Milk Exchange List is divided according to fat content. Only skim milk products are nonfat. To use lowfat and whole milk products, subtract appropriate Fat Exchanges. At least half the fat contained in lowfat and whole milk is saturated.

fat exchange

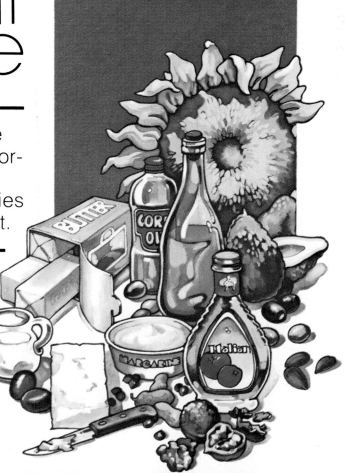

Fats (page 30) can be a deceptive group of foods. They pack lots of calories into beguilingly small parcels. Often hidden in foods, fats add calories and extra pounds before you know it.

Fats provide energy and ward off hunger sensations. They give us essential fatty acids, fat-soluble vitamins, and calories. Because all fats are concentrated calorie sources, measure foods on this list carefully.

Note that the Fat Exchange List designates saturated, and unsaturated fats. Dietary saturated fats tend to raise the level of blood cholesterol in some people.

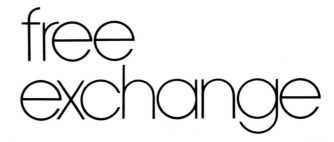

free exchange

The only limit on Free Exchanges (page 30) is your appetite. They are insignificant in terms of calories.

Use the Free Exchanges to add the gourmet touches that make your meals as pleasant and attractive to serve as they are to eat. Use herbs and spices freely to pep up your palate.

Non-caloric sweetener should be used only in moderate amounts in place of sugar. It's available in liquid, tablet, and powdered form.

alcohol calories do count

No matter what wishful thinkers say, alcohol calories count the same as others. In fact, alcohol contains more calories per ounce than proteins or carbohydrates and nearly as many as fats. Alcohol calories can be tempting, so weight watchers beware.

A balanced reducing diet furnishes essential nutrients. Therefore, foods should never be subtracted from a reducing diet to make room for alcohol calories. The calories of an alcoholic beverage should be *added to* the calories of a reducing diet. This slows the speed of the reducing diet and indeed impedes progress.

Discover how quickly alcohol can add unwanted calories to a reducing diet as you compare these figures for various alcoholic beverages. One eight-ounce glass of beer provides about 114 calories. A three-ounce daiquiri supplies about 122 calories, and a 10-ounce tom collins supplies about 180 calories. One jigger (one and one-half ounces) of 90-proof rum, vodka, gin, or whiskey supplies about 110 calories.

Dry wines contain fewer calories than the sweet wines. Table wines containing less than 15% alcohol provide about 87 calories in each glass of three and one-half ounces. Table wines include those such as burgundy, chablis, champagne, chianti, claret, rhine, rosé, and sauterne. Dessert wines containing more than 15% alcohol provide about 81 calories per two-ounce glass. Included in the dessert wine category are sherry, port, and vermouth.

Alcohol can be used *in moderation for cooking purposes*. Most of the calories from alcohol are burned off quickly when heated, leaving only its subtle flavor behind. Add a dash of dry wine to some of your longstanding recipes for new aroma and flavor.

food exchange lists

meat

LEAN MEAT EXCHANGE	Each serving below is based on cooked meat with fat trimmed. One Exchange provides seven grams protein, three grams fat, and 55 calories. Most Exchanges except shellfish are fairly low in saturated fat and cholesterol.		
beef: 1 ounce	dried beef flank steak tripe	sirloin tenderloin chuck	plate spareribs plate short ribs round, bottom or top	plate skirt steak all cuts rump
lamb: 1 ounce	shank leg	rib shoulder	sirloin	loin

pork:
1 ounce
	leg (whole rump,
	       center shank)
		fully cooked ham
		   (center slices)		

veal: 1 ounce	leg shoulder	loin cutlets	rib	shank
fish: fresh, canned, or frozen	bass (1 oz.) carp (1 oz.) catfish (1 oz.) cod (1 oz.) eel (1 oz.) flounder (1 oz.) haddock (1 oz.) hake (1 oz.)	halibut (1 oz.) herring (1 oz.) mackerel (¼ cup) mullet (1 oz.) pike (1 oz.) pollock (1 oz.) pompano (1 oz.) red snapper (1 oz.)	rockfish (1 oz.) salmon (1 oz.) (¼ cup, canned) sardines (3) smelt (1 oz.) sole (1 oz.) swordfish (1 oz.) tuna (¼ cup)	whitefish (1 oz.) perch (1 oz.) clams (1 oz.) crab (¼ cup) oysters (1 oz.) scallops (1 oz.) shrimp (1 oz.) lobster (¼ cup)
poultry: without skin 1 ounce		Cornish hen turkey	pheasant chicken	Guinea hen

cheeses containing less
   than 5% butterfat
1 ounce
	cottage cheese, dry
	   and 2% butterfat
	¼ cup
		dried beans and peas
		   (omit 1 Bread Exchange)
		½ cup cooked	

MEDIUM-FAT MEAT EXCHANGE

Each serving is based on cooked meat and counts as one Medium-Fat Meat Exchange. Because of their higher fat content, Medium-Fat Meat Exchanges count as one Lean Meat Exchange and one-half Fat Exchange on the Daily Meal Plans. One Medium-Fat Meat Exchange supplies seven grams protein, five and one-half grams fat, and 75 calories. Only peanut butter is low in saturated fat and cholesterol.

beef: 1 ounce	ground beef (15% fat)	ground round (commercial)	corned beef (canned)	rib eye steak
pork: 1 ounce	loin (all cuts tenderloin) boiled ham	shoulder arm picnic	shoulder blade Boston roast	Canadian-style bacon
variety meat—beef, veal, pork, or lamb: 1 ounce (high in cholesterol)	heart liver	sweetbreads	kidney
cheese:	mozzarella ricotta 1 ounce	parmesan 3 tbsp.	farmer's cheese 1 ounce	neufchatel 1 ounce
cottage cheese, creamed ¼ cup	**egg** (high in cholesterol) 1	**peanut butter** (omit 2 additional Fat Exchanges) 2 tbsp.	

HIGH-FAT MEAT EXCHANGE

Each serving below is based on cooked meat and counts as one High-Fat Meat Exchange. Because of their high fat content, foods in this Exchange List count as one Lean Meat Exchange and one Fat Exchange. One High-Fat Meat Exchange supplies seven grams of protein, eight grams of fat, and 100 calories.

beef: 1 ounce	brisket corned beef brisket	ground beef (more than 20% fat) hamburger (commercial)	ground chuck (commercial)	rib roast rib steak top loin steak
lamb: 1 ounce	breast		**veal:** 1 ounce	breast
pork: 1 ounce	spareribs loin back ribs	ground pork deviled ham	cook-before-eating ham (country-style)	
poultry: 1 ounce	capon	duck (domestic)	goose	
cheese: cheddar types 1 ounce	**cold cuts** 4½ x ⅛-inch slice	**frankfurter** 1 small	

bread

Each serving of the following breads, cereals, crackers, dried beans, starchy vegetables, and prepared foods counts as one Bread Exchange. All items except those listed as prepared foods are lowfat. Be sure to charge yourself for the extra Fat Exchanges contained in the prepared foods. One Bread Exchange provides two grams of protein, 15 grams of carbohydrate, and 70 calories.

bread:

white, whole wheat, French, Italian, rye, pumpernickel, or raisin	1 slice	bagel, small	½	hamburger bun	½
		English muffin, small	½	dried bread crumbs	3 tbsp.
		plain dinner roll	1	tortilla, 6 inch	1
		frankfurter bun	½		

cereal:

bran flakes	½ cup	cooked cereal	½ cup	popcorn (popped, no fat added)	3 cups
other ready-to-eat unsweetened cereal	¾ cup	cooked grits	½ cup	cornmeal (dry)	2 tbsp.
		cooked rice or barley	½ cup	flour	2½ tbsp.
puffed cereal (unfrosted)	1 cup	cooked pasta, macaroni, or noodles	½ cup	wheat germ	¼ cup

crackers:

arrowroot	3	pretzels, 3⅛x⅛ inch	25	saltines	6
graham, 2½ inch	2	rye wafers, 3½x2 inch	3	soda, 2½-inch square	4
matzo, 6x4 inch	½				
oyster	20				

beans, peas, and lentils:

		beans, peas, lentils (dried, cooked) (omit 1 Lean Meat Exchange)	½ cup	baked beans, no pork (canned)	¼ cup

starchy vegetables:

corn	⅓ cup	peas (canned or frozen)	½ cup	pumpkin	¾ cup
corn on cob	1 small			winter squash	½ cup
lima beans	½ cup	potato (white)	1 small	yam or sweet potato	¼ cup
parsnips	⅔ cup	potato (mashed)	½ cup		

prepared foods:

muffin, plain small (omit 1 Fat Exchange)	1	potatoes, French-fried (omit 1 Fat Exchange)	8	potato or corn chips (omit 2 Fat Exchanges)	15
pancake, 5x½ inch (omit 1 Fat Exchange)	1	waffle, 5x½ inch (omit 1 Fat Exchange)	1	corn muffin, 2 inch (omit 1 Fat Exchange)	1
biscuit, 2-inch diameter (omit 1 Fat Exchange)	1	corn bread, 2x2x1 inch (omit 1 Fat Exchange)	1	crackers, round butter type (omit 1 Fat Exchange)	5

fruit

The amount of each fruit listed (with no sugar added) counts as one Fruit Exchange. Fruits are nonfat. One Exchange contains 10 grams carbohydrate and 40 calories.

apple	1 small	figs, fresh or dried	1	orange juice	½ cup
apple juice or cider	⅓ cup	grapefruit	½	papaya	¾ cup
applesauce		grapefruit juice	½ cup	peach	1 medium
(unsweetened)	½ cup	grapes	12	pear	1 small
apricots, fresh	2 medium	grape juice	¼ cup	persimmon, native	1 medium
apricots, dried	4 halves	mango	½ small	pineapple	½ cup
banana	½ small	melon		pineapple juice	⅓ cup
berries		cantaloupe	¼ small	plums	2 medium
strawberries	¾ cup	honeydew	⅛ medium	prunes	2 medium
other berries	½ cup	watermelon	1 cup	prune juice	¼ cup
cherries	10 large	nectarine	1 small	raisins	2 tbsp.
cranberries	as desired	orange	1 small	tangerine	1 medium
dates	2				

vegetable

Each half-cup serving counts as one Exchange and provides two grams protein, five grams carbohydrate, and 25 calories. Vegetables are nonfat. Free vegetables are listed below and in the Free List.

asparagus	brussels sprouts	eggplant	rutabaga	tomato juice
beans, green	cabbage	mushrooms	sauerkraut	turnips
or yellow	carrots	okra	spinach and	vegetable juice
bean sprouts	cauliflower	onions	other greens	cocktail
beets	celery	peppers	summer squash	zucchini
broccoli	cucumbers	rhubarb	tomatoes	

The following raw vegetables are all Free Exchanges and may be eaten in any amounts:	chicory	escarole	radishes
	Chinese cabbage	lettuce	watercress
	endive	parsley	

milk

Milk Exchanges are shown below. Lowfat and whole milk products cost extra Fat Exchanges. One Exchange equals eight grams protein, 12 grams carbohydrate, and 80 calories.

nonfat fortified milk:	skim or nonfat milk	1 cup	canned evaporated skim milk	½ cup
	nonfat dry milk powder	⅓ cup		
	yogurt, made from skim milk (plain)	1 cup	buttermilk, made from skim milk	1 cup
lowfat fortified milk:	1% fat milk (omit ½ Fat Exchange)	1 cup	yogurt, made from 2% milk (plain) (omit 1 Fat Exchange)	¾ cup
	2% fat milk (omit 1 Fat Exchange)	1 cup		
whole milk (omit 2 Fat Exchanges):	whole milk	1 cup	canned evaporated whole milk	½ cup
	yogurt, made from whole milk (plain)	1 cup	buttermilk, made from whole milk	1 cup

fat

Fats below are designated as saturated, monounsaturated, or polyunsaturated. Saturated fats are found primarily in animal food products and are believed to raise the level of cholesterol in the blood, a risk factor associated with heart disease. Heart specialists recommend substituting the unsaturated fats for the saturated fats in the diet whenever possible. Vegetable oils such as corn, cottonseed, safflower, soybean, and sunflower are low in saturated fats. The fats listed below are saturated unless marked with an asterisk (*). One asterisk (*) indicates a fat content that is primarily monounsaturated. Two asterisks (**) indicate a fat content that is primarily polyunsaturated, while three asterisks (***) indicate a polyunsaturated fat content only if the product is made with corn, cottonseed, safflower, soy, or sunflower oil. One Fat Exchange provides five grams of fat and 45 calories.

avocado* (4-inch diameter)	⅛	cream cheese	1 tbsp.	margarine, regular	1 tsp.
		Italian salad dressing***	1 tbsp.	lard	1 tsp.
bacon, crisp-cooked	1 slice	French salad dressing***	1 tbsp.	mayonnaise***	1 tsp.
bacon fat	1 tsp.			olives*	5 small
butter	1 tsp.	margarine,*** soft (tub or stick)	1 tsp.	salad dressing,*** mayonnaise-type	2 tsp.
cream, light	2 tbsp.				
cream, sour	2 tbsp.				
cream, whipping	1 tbsp.			salt pork	¾-in. cube

nuts:

almonds*	10 whole	peanuts*		walnuts**	6 small
pecans*	2 large whole	Spanish	20 whole	other*	6 small
		Virginia	10 whole		

oil:

1 tsp.	corn**	safflower**	sunflower**	peanut*
	cottonseed**	soy**	olive*	

free

Listed below are flavor bonuses with Free Exchange ratings. Also included on this list are raw vegetables which can be eaten in any amount desired.

salt	vinegar	low-calorie carbonated beverages	unflavored gelatin	endive
pepper	mustard			escarole
herbs	tea		unsweetened pickles	lettuce
spices	coffee	low-calorie flavored gelatin		parsley
lemon	nonfat bouillon		chicory	radishes
lime	non-caloric sweetener		Chinese cabbage	watercress
horseradish				

Food Exchange Lists (pages 26-30) are based on material in the booklet *Exchange Lists for Meal Planning* prepared by committees of the American Diabetes Association, Inc. and the American Dietetic Association.

exchange lists for packaged foods

No need to be frustrated by packaged convenience foods. Use the Exchange Lists for Packaged Foods to fit them into your Daily Meal Plan. Because packaged foods are so diverse, they're identified by brand. Unless noted, Exchanges are based on products prepared according to package directions.

Main dishes	Serving size	Exchanges per serving
Morningstar Farms®		
breakfast patties	2 patties	2⅓ lean meat + ⅓ bread + 1½ fat
breakfast strips	3 strips	½ lean meat + 1¾ fat
breakfast links	3 links	2 lean meat + 1½ fat
luncheon slices	2 slices	1 lean meat + ⅓ bread
Swift		
Sizzlean® pork breakfast strips	2 strips	1 lean meat + 1 fat
Swanson® frozen entrées		
chicken nibbles with French fries	6 ounces	2 lean meat + 2 bread + 3 fat
English style (fish and chips)	5 ounces	2 lean meat + 1½ bread + 2 fat
fried chicken with whipped potatoes	7 ounces	2 lean meat + 2 bread + 2 fat
gravy and sliced beef with whipped potatoes	8 ounces	1 lean meat + 1½ bread + 1 fat
salisbury steak with crinkle-cut potatoes	5½ ounces	2 lean meat + 2 bread + 3 fat
spaghetti with breaded veal	8¼ ounces	1 lean meat + 2 bread + 2 fat
French toast with sausages	4½ ounces	2 lean meat + 2 bread + 1 fat

Main dishes *continued*	Serving size	Exchanges per serving
Dinty Moore®		
beef stew	7½ ounces	1½ lean meat + ½ bread + 1 vegetable + 1 fat
noodles and chicken	7½ ounces	1 lean meat + 1 bread + 2 fat
Heinz		
chicken stew with dumplings	7¼ ounces	1 lean meat + 1 bread + 1 vegetable + 1 fat
macaroni in cheese sauce	7½ ounces	1 lean meat + 1½ bread + ½ fat
noodles and tuna	7½ ounces	1 lean meat + 1 bread + 1 vegetable
noodles with beef and sauce	7½ ounces	1 lean meat + 1 bread + ½ fat
spaghetti in tomato sauce with cheese	7½ ounces	2 bread + ½ fat
spaghetti with meat sauce	7¼ ounces	½ lean meat + 1 bread + 1 vegetable + 1 fat
Kraft®		
macaroni and cheese dinner	¾ cup	½ lean meat + 2 bread + 2½ fat
American-style spaghetti dinner	1 cup	3 bread + 1 fat
Mrs. Paul's® Kitchens, Inc.		
frozen deviled crab cakes	1 cake	1 lean meat + 1 bread + 1 fat
frozen fish sticks	4 sticks	1 lean meat + 1 bread + 4 fat

Meal accompaniments	Serving size	Exchanges per serving
Stove Top® (prepared with butter or margarine)		
stuffing mix	½ cup	1½ bread + 2 fat
Betty Crocker®		
noodles almondine	¼ package	2 bread + 2 fat
noodles Romanoff	¼ package	1 bread + ½ milk + 2 fat
Green Giant® Bake N' Serve frozen vegetables		
broccoli in cheese sauce	3½ ounces	1 vegetable + 1 fat

Meal accompaniments *continued*	Serving size	Exchanges per serving

Green Giant® Bake N' Serve frozen vegetables *continued*

cauliflower in cheese sauce	3½ ounces	1 vegetable + 1 fat
creamed peas	3½ ounces	1 bread + 1 fat

La Choy® frozen vegetables (without added butter or margarine)

Chinese vegetables	3.3 ounces	1 vegetable
pea pods	1½ ounces	1 vegetable

Birdseye® frozen vegetables (without added butter or margarine)

Bavarian-style beans with spaetzle	3.3 ounces	2 vegetable
Danish-style vegetables	3.3 ounces	1 vegetable
Italian-style vegetables	3.3 ounces	½ bread
Japanese-style vegetables	3.3 ounces	1 vegetable

Soups	Serving size	Exchanges per serving

Lipton® Cup-a-Soup (1 serving size; prepared with water)

bean	6 ounces	½ lean meat + 1 bread
beef-flavored noodle	6 ounces	½ bread
vegetable beef	6 ounces	1 vegetable
cream-style chicken	6 ounces	⅔ bread + 1 fat
cream of mushroom	6 ounces	⅔ bread + 1 fat
cream of tomato	6 ounces	1 bread + ½ fat
spring vegetable	6 ounces	2 vegetable
chicken noodle with meat	6 ounces	½ bread

Nestle® Souptime® (1 serving size; prepared with water)

chicken noodle	6 ounces	½ bread
beef noodle	6 ounces	½ bread
cream of chicken	6 ounces	⅔ bread + 1 fat
tomato	6 ounces	1 bread
French onion	6 ounces	1 vegetable
green pea	6 ounces	½ lean meat + 1 bread
mushroom	6 ounces	⅔ bread + 1 fat
cream of vegetable	6 ounces	1½ vegetable + 1 fat

34

Soups *continued*	Serving size	Exchanges per serving
Campbell's® condensed (prepared with water)		
cheddar cheese	11 ounces	1 milk + 3 fat
chicken noodle	10 ounces	1 bread
chicken with rice	10 ounces	1 bread
cream of mushroom	10 ounces	1 bread + 2 fat
clam chowder, Manhattan	10 ounces	1 bread + ½ fat
minestrone	10 ounces	1 bread + ½ fat
onion	10 ounces	1 bread
tomato	10 ounces	1 bread + 1 vegetable
vegetable	10 ounces	1 bread + 1 vegetable
vegetarian vegetable	10 ounces	1 bread

Breads	Serving size	Exchanges per serving
Ortega®		
taco shell	1 shell	1 bread
Pepperidge Farm®		
very thin bread—white	2 slices	1 bread
very thin bread—whole wheat	2 slices	1 bread
croutons—cheddar cheese, seasoned, onion-garlic, or plain	½ cup	1½ bread + 1 fat
croutons—cheese-garlic	½ cup	1 bread + 1½ fat
Pillsbury®		
refrigerated plain buttermilk biscuits	2 biscuits	1½ bread
refrigerated butterflake dinner rolls	1 roll	1 bread + ½ fat
refrigerated crescent dinner rolls	1 roll	1 bread + 1 fat
bread mixes—applesauce, apricot-nut, banana, blueberry-nut, cranberry, date, or nut	1/16 loaf	1½ bread + ½ fat
hot roll mix	2 rolls	2 bread + 1 fat
Sara Lee®		
croissant rolls	1 roll	1 bread + 1 fat
parkerhouse rolls	1 roll	1 bread + ½ fat

Breads continued	Serving size	Exchanges per serving
Sarah Lee® continued		
poppy seed rolls	1 roll	½ bread + ½ fat

Miscellaneous	Serving size	Exchanges per serving
Contadina® or Hunt's®		
pizza sauce	1 cup	1½ bread + 1 fat
tomato sauce	1 cup	1 bread
tomato paste	¾ cup	2 bread
Dannon® yogurt		
flavored—coffee, lemon, or vanilla	8 ounces	1½ bread + 1 milk + ½ fat
fruit—strawberry, cherry, honey, etc.	8 ounces	1 bread + 2 fruit + 1 milk + ½ fat
Kraft®		
soft Diet Parkay® imitation margarine	1 tbsp.	1 fat
zesty Italian low-calorie salad dressing	2 tbsp.	free
French-style low-calorie salad dressing	2 tbsp.	¼ bread + 1 fat
Dia-Mel®		
whipped mayonnaise-type salad dressing substitute	2 tbsp.	1 fat
Borden®		
Lite-line® pasteurized process cheese product	1 ounce	1 lean meat
General Foods Products		
Jell-O® brand pudding and pie filling (prepared with nonfat milk)	½ cup	1½ bread + ½ milk
Jell-O® brand cheesecake	⅛ cake	2½ bread + 2 fat
Jell-O® brand egg custard (prepared with nonfat milk)	½ cup	1 bread + ½ milk
D-Zerta® low-calorie pudding (prepared with nonfat milk)	½ cup	½ bread + ½ milk
D-Zerta® low-calorie whipped topping	3 tbsp.	½ fat

daily meal plans

FOOD EXCHANGES AND COLOR SYMBOLS		1,000 cal. per day	1,200 cal. per day	1,500 cal. per day
		no. of Exchanges	no. of Exchanges	no. of Exchanges
breakfast	Lean Meat Exchange	1	1	2
	Bread Exchange	1	1	2
	Fruit Exchange	1	1	1
	Milk Exchange	½	½	½
	Fat Exchange	1	2	2
	Free Exchange	as desired	as desired	as desired
lunch	Lean Meat Exchange	2	2	2
	Bread Exchange	1	1	2
	Fruit Exchange	1	1	1
	Vegetable Exchange	1	2	2
	Milk Exchange	1	1	1
	Fat Exchange	1	1	2
	Free Exchange	as desired	as desired	as desired
dinner	Lean Meat Exchange	2	4	4
	Bread Exchange	1	1	1
	Fruit Exchange	1	1	1
	Vegetable Exchange	1	2	2
	Milk Exchange	½	½	½
	Fat Exchange	2	2	3
	Free Exchange	as desired	as desired	as desired

Planning diet menus isn't difficult if you use the Food Exchanges to guide you. Choose a meal plan giving a daily calorie deficit that lets you reduce no more than two pounds a week (see pages 9-11). Follow the food allotments in your Daily Meal Plan and make menu selections from the Food Exchange Lists (see pages 26-35) and the recipe section.

menu planning steps

Menu planning can be fun, especially when you don't have to count calories. The Daily Meal Plans (page 36) and the Food Exchange Lists (pages 26-35) are the working tools.

Decide on the Daily Meal Plan that helps you lose no more than two pounds per week. Follow your Meal Plan and make menu selections from the Food Exchange Lists and recipes in this book.

Use the following Menu Planning Steps: (They were used to plan the tasty dinner menu at right from the 1,200-calorie meal plan for dinner.)

1. Choose a main dish. It may be strictly meat or it may be a combination of Exchanges. Four ounces of broiled sirloin steak represent four Lean Meat Exchanges, the exact Meat Exchange allowance.
2. Select a Bread Exchange. One small baked potato equals one Bread Exchange.
3. Decide on a Fruit Exchange as a meal accompaniment or dessert. Tapioca Pudding Parfait is the dessert in this menu. The recipe and Exchange values can be found in the recipe section. One serving supplies one-half Milk Exchange in addition to one Fruit Exchange.
4. Pick compatible vegetables. Two Exchanges are allowed. Tangy Vegetable Vinaigrette, found in recipe section, and one-half cup of cooked carrots account for the two Exchanges.
5. Add any Milk Exchanges not used in cooking. Because one-half Milk Exchange was used for the Tapioca Pudding Parfait, there's no need to add milk here.
6. Decide on any Fat Exchanges not used in cooking. Two tablespoons of dairy sour cream on the potato account for one Fat Exchange, while one tablespoon of diet imitation margarine on the carrots equals the remaining Fat Exchange.
7. Add Free Exchanges to round out the meal. Have coffee or tea to accompany dessert.

meal plan

- 4 Lean Meat Exchanges
- 1 Bread Exchange
- 1 Fruit Exchange
- 2 Vegetable Exchanges
- ½ Milk Exchange
- 2 Fat Exchanges
- Free Exchanges

menu

- 4 ounces broiled sirloin steak
- 1 small baked potato
- 2 tbsp. dairy sour cream
- Tangy Vegetable Vinaigrette*
- ½ cup cooked sliced carrots
- 1 tbsp. diet imitation margarine
- Tapioca Pudding Parfait*
- coffee or tea

* see recipe section

1,000 calorie menus

Can the famished reducer really appease his appetite with only 1,000 calories a day? You bet. We have created three satisfying menus that provide only 1,000 calories to show that dieters, too, can enjoy hearty, flavorful foods. The seven easy Menu Planning Steps on page 37 were used to create the menus. Take a closer look and you'll discover some meals use extra Exchanges while others are missing an Exchange or two. Don't be mystified.

The Exchanges simply have been moved from one meal to another. Foods marked with an asterisk (*) are in the recipe section. Don't cut back to fewer than 1,000 calories daily. Check to make sure you lose no more than two pounds a week.

menu planning tips

Wake up to a slice of crisp toast topped with a layer of bubbly-hot cheddar cheese. Fresh blackberries and skim milk round out breakfast with one-half Bread Exchange left over. Don't worry, you'll find a good use for that extra Exchange at dinner. Lunch features healthful Vegetarian Sprout

Sandwiches with fresh avocado and a side dish of cottage cheese served on a lettuce-lined plate. You may want to add a few radish slices to the cottage cheese for color—they're free. The dinner menu is pictured above. Fruited Lamb Chops team up with broccoli spears and almond-studded rice for a satisfying meal. The four teaspoons of sliced almonds (or 10 whole almonds) equal one Fat Exchange. We've borrowed that extra one-half Bread Exchange from breakfast so you can top off dinner with an icy Banana Freeze.

breakfast

DAILY MEAL PLAN	MENU A

DAILY MEAL PLAN

- 1 Lean Meat Exchange
- 1 Bread Exchange
- 1 Fruit Exchange
- ½ Milk Exchange
- 1 Fat Exchange
- Free Exchanges

MENU A

1 slice broiled cheese
 toast made with:
- 1 oz. cheddar cheese
- 1 slice very thin bread
- ½ cup fresh blackberries
- ½ cup skim milk

Exchanges not used:
- ½ Bread Exchange

lunch

DAILY MEAL PLAN

- 2 Lean Meat Exchanges
- 1 Bread Exchange
- 1 Fruit Exchange
- 1 Vegetable Exchange
- 1 Milk Exchange
- 1 Fat Exchange
- Free Exchanges

MENU A

Vegetarian Sprout Sandwiches*
- ⅛ avocado, sliced
- ¼ cup lowfat cottage cheese (no more than 2% butterfat) on lettuce-lined plate
- 1 small apple
- 1 cup skim milk
- coffee or tea

dinner

DAILY MEAL PLAN

- 2 Lean Meat Exchanges
- 1 Bread Exchange
- 1 Fruit Exchange
- 1 Vegetable Exchange
- ½ Milk Exchange
- 2 Fat Exchanges
- Free Exchanges

MENU A

Fruited Lamb Chops*
- ½ cup cooked rice with 4 tsp. sliced almonds (10 whole)
- ½ cup cooked broccoli
- 1½ tsp. diet imitation margarine
- Banana Freeze*
- ½ cup skim milk
- coffee or tea

Extra Exchanges used:
- ½ Bread Exchange

breakfast

	DAILY MEAL PLAN		MENU B
●	1 Lean Meat Exchange	●◖	1 soft-cooked egg
●	1 Bread Exchange	●	1 slice raisin toast
○	1 Fruit Exchange	◖	1½ tsp. diet imitation
◖	½ Milk Exchange		margarine
●	1 Fat Exchange	○	⅓ cup apple juice
●	Free Exchanges	◖	½ cup skim milk

lunch

●●	2 Lean Meat Exchanges	●◖ ◖	Trimming Tuna Toss*
●	1 Bread Exchange	●	1 slice rye bread
○	1 Fruit Exchange	●	1 tbsp. cream cheese
●	1 Vegetable Exchange	◖	¼ cup carrot sticks
●	1 Milk Exchange	○	1 medium peach
●	1 Fat Exchange	●	1 cup skim milk
●	Free Exchanges		
			Exchanges not used:
		◖	½ Lean Meat Exchange

dinner

●●	2 Lean Meat Exchanges	●●◖	No Crust Pizza*
●	1 Bread Exchange	●●	
○	1 Fruit Exchange	◖	1 slice very thin bread
●	1 Vegetable Exchange	○◖	Zippy Waldorf Salad*
◖	½ Milk Exchange	◖◖	½ cup low-calorie choco-
●●	2 Fat Exchanges		late-flavored pudding
●	Free Exchanges	◖	3 tbsp. low-calorie
			whipped dessert
			topping
			Extra Exchanges used:
		◖	½ Lean Meat Exchange

MENU C

● ◖ 1 egg omelet, made with

◖   1½ tsp. diet imitation

      margarine

● 1 cup puffed rice cereal

◖ ½ cup skim milk

○ ½ small banana, sliced

● coffee or tea

---

   1 roast beef sandwich, made with

● ●   2 oz. cooked lean roast beef

●   2 slices very thin white bread

●   1 tbsp. diet imitation

      margarine

●   lettuce

● ½ cup vegetable relishes

○ 1 small orange

● 1 cup skim milk

● coffee or tea

● ● ● Turkey Asparagus Pilaf*

● ●

● mixed salad greens

● 2 tbsp. low-calorie Italian

   salad dressing (no more than

   8 calories per tablespoon)

○ ● Plum Whip*

◖ ½ cup skim milk

● coffee or tea

menu planning tips

Egg, raisin toast, diet imitation margarine, apple juice, and skim milk combine to make breakfast in Menu B. Rye bread spread with cream cheese accents the Trimming Tuna Toss at lunch. Add carrot sticks, a peach, and a glass of skim milk and you ease those hunger pangs and still have one-half Lean Meat Exchange left for dinner. No Crust Pizza adds an Italian flair to a dinner that's suitable for the whole family. And what a surprise: chocolate pudding with whipped topping for dessert (low-calorie, of course).

Menu C features a hefty breakfast composed of an omelet and cereal topped with banana slices. Good news for the dieter: It uses only those Exchanges allowed for breakfast on the 1,000-calorie Daily Meal Plan. The roast beef sandwich for lunch makes a hearty entrée. Be sure to use roast beef from the Lean Meat Exchange only. Very thin bread and diet imitation margarine (found in the Food Exchange Lists for Packaged Foods on pages 31-35) help stretch the lunchtime Bread and Fat Exchanges. Choose vegetable relishes from the Vegetable Exchange List. Raw broccoli, carrots, cauliflowerets, celery, cucumbers, and mushrooms are among the possibilities. Round out the meal with an orange and a glass of skim milk. For dinner, Turkey Asparagus Pilaf is practically a meal in itself. It supplies all the Meat, Bread, Vegetable, and half the Fat Exchanges for the entire dinner. Mixed salad greens (chicory, Chinese cabbage, endive, escarole, lettuce, parsley, and watercress —take your choice) are free. So is the two-tablespoon serving of Italian salad dressing, as long as it provides no more than 8 calories per tablespoon. Read the label carefully; it states the calorie content. Any meal goes better when you include a dessert like Plum Whip. Add one-half cup of skim milk and your choice of coffee or tea, and you've satisfied your appetite *and* the Exchange requirements for the 1,000-calorie Daily Meal Plan.

*see recipe section

1,200 calorie menus

Has dieting got you down? Our 1,200-calorie reducing menus will banish boredom from your diet with an array of imaginative ideas and robust recipes. To create these diet menus, we have applied the seven Menu Planning Steps found on page 37. When you compare the menus to the 1,200-calorie Daily Meal Plan, you will discover that some meals appear to use an extra Exchange or two, while other meals are "short" Exchanges. To trace the moving Exchanges, we've used the headlines "Extra Exchanges used" and "Exchanges not used." Asterisk (*) denotes the foods that are found in the recipe section.

menu planning tips

A well-balanced breakfast highlighted with fresh raspberries starts the dieter's day. The luncheon (pictured above) includes Confetti Cheese Quiche, pea pods, apple slices, and a salad accented with radish slices. This light tasting lunch saves you one Lean Meat Exchange for dinner, when you capitalize on Beef Burgundy with rice, cut green beans, and a peach half topped with one-half cup cottage cheese. Don't let this shift of Food Exchanges from lunch to dinner confuse you. As long as the daily *total* of Food Exchanges remains the same as those allowed on the 1,200-calorie Daily Meal Plan, you can consume the Exchanges whenever you please—morning, afternoon, or night. Coffee, tea, and low-calorie carbonated beverages are all Free Exchanges and can be added any time of the day.

breakfast.

DAILY MEAL PLAN	MENU A
1 Lean Meat Exchange	1 egg, fried in 1 tbsp.
1 Bread Exchange	diet imitation margarine
1 Fruit Exchange	½ small bagel, toasted
½ Milk Exchange	1½ tsp. diet imitation
2 Fat Exchanges	margarine
Free Exchanges	½ cup fresh raspberries
	½ cup skim milk

lunch

	MENU A
2 Lean Meat Exchanges	Confetti Cheese Quiche*
1 Bread Exchange	1½ ounces cooked pea pods
1 Fruit Exchange	mixed salad greens
2 Vegetable Exchanges	Tangy Tomato Dressing*
1 Milk Exchange	1 small apple, sliced
1 Fat Exchange	1 cup skim milk
Free Exchanges	coffee or tea

Exchanges not used:
1 Lean Meat Exchange

dinner

	MENU A
4 Lean Meat Exchanges	Beef Burgundy*
1 Bread Exchange	
1 Fruit Exchange	½ cup cooked cut green beans
2 Vegetable Exchanges	1 tbsp. diet imitation margarine
½ Milk Exchange	1 medium peach, halved
2 Fat Exchanges	½ cup lowfat cottage cheese (no more than 2% butterfat)
Free Exchanges	½ cup skim milk
	coffee or tea

Extra Exchanges used:
1 Lean Meat Exchange

breakfast

DAILY MEAL PLAN	MENU B
● 1 Lean Meat Exchange	● 1 1-oz. fully cooked center-cut ham slice
● 1 Bread Exchange	●● 1 5-inch pancake
○ 1 Fruit Exchange	○ ½ cup blueberries
◐ ½ Milk Exchange	◐ ½ cup skim milk
●● 2 Fat Exchanges	● coffee or tea
● Free Exchanges	

Exchanges not used:

● 1 Fat Exchange

lunch

DAILY MEAL PLAN	MENU B
●● 2 Lean Meat Exchanges	●●● Corned Beef Slaw-Wiches*
● 1 Bread Exchange	◐●●
○ 1 Fruit Exchange	●◐ ¾ cup vegetable relishes
●● 2 Vegetable Exchanges	○ ½ cup unsweetened applesauce
● 1 Milk Exchange	● 1 cup skim milk
● 1 Fat Exchange	
● Free Exchanges	

Extra Exchanges used:

● 1 Fat Exchange

dinner

DAILY MEAL PLAN	MENU B
●●●● 4 Lean Meat Exchanges	● Icy Tomato Tune-Up*
● 1 Bread Exchange	●●●● Lemon Poached Salmon*
○ 1 Fruit Exchange	◐ Tartar Sauce*
●● 2 Vegetable Exchanges	● ½ cup cooked cut asparagus
◐ ½ Milk Exchange	●● 1 refrigerated crescent roll
●● 2 Fat Exchanges	○ Ruby Fruit Compote*
● Free Exchanges	◐ 1 tbsp. dairy sour cream
	◐ ½ cup skim milk

MENU C
- ●◖ 1 hard-cooked egg
- ●◖ 1½ slices cooked bacon
- ◐ ¼ small cantaloupe with lime
- ● Mexican-Style Hot Chocolate*

Extra Exchanges used:
- ◖ ½ Milk Exchange

Exchanges not used:
- ● 1 Bread Exchange

- ●●●◖● Turkey Asparagus Stacks*
- ●◖
- ● Herbed Tomato Soup*
- ◐◖● Pineapple Dream Pie*
- ● iced tea

Extra Exchanges used:
- ◖ ½ Lean Meat Exchange
- ◖ ½ Fat Exchange

Exchanges not used:
- ◖ ½ Milk Exchange

- ●●●◖ Taco Compuesto*
- ●●●●
- ●◖
- ◐◖ Tapioca Pudding Parfait*

Extra Exchanges used:
- ● 1 Bread Exchange

Exchanges not used:
- ◖ ½ Lean Meat Exchange
- ◖ ½ Fat Exchange

menu planning tips

Menu B features ham, a blueberry-topped pancake, and skim milk for breakfast. Be sure to use fully cooked center-cut ham slices and *not* boiled ham, because there's a difference of one-half Fat Exchange. Always conserve if possible. Top the pancake with one-half cup of juicy blueberries and eliminate the need for butter or margarine. The Fat Exchange you save is used at lunch so you can enjoy the Corned Beef Slaw-Wiches. Vegetable relishes (your choice of any of the Vegetable Exchanges served raw), applesauce, and skim milk complete the lunch menu. The Icy Tomato Tune-Up will prime your appetite for dinner. Or, if you can't wait, enjoy Icy Tomato Tune-Up as a mid-afternoon snack. Lemon Poached Salmon pairs up with a creamy Tartar Sauce at dinner. For the finale serve refreshing Ruby Fruit Compote.

Menu C, pictured on the cover, is a bit more complicated than some of the other menus. We've dropped a few Exchanges here and added other Exchanges there to bring you an imaginative menu. Trace the Food Exchanges and tally the totals. Here are the menu mechanics:

By saying no to the breadbasket in the morning, you can indulge in *two* tacos at dinner. So you won't feel shortchanged at breakfast, we've borrowed one-half Milk Exchange from lunch to make room for a steaming mug of Mexican-Style Hot Chocolate. The main luncheon dish, Turkey Asparagus Stacks, uses extra Lean Meat and Fat Exchanges from dinner. But you won't notice the missing Exchanges at dinner when you treat yourself to Taco Compuesto. If you think it's a case of "musical Exchanges," you're right, but it offers a lot of eating satisfaction for only 1,200 calories.

*see recipe section

1,500 calorie menus

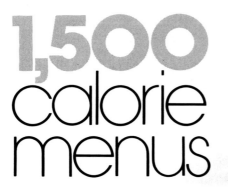

The hearty 1,500-calorie menus offer more flavorful foods than you ever thought you'd be eating on a diet. Although the menus offer a lot of eating satisfaction, reducing speed will be slower than that produced by 1,000- or 1,200-calorie menus. The seven Menu Planning Steps on page 37 were used to create the menu ideas. They're the same seven steps you will use to plan your own imaginative menus. Remember that it's possible to move Exchanges or "save" Exchanges to snack on later that day or night as long as the daily total of Exchanges remains the same. Foods marked with an asterisk (*) are in the recipe section of this book.

menu planning tips

The eye-opening breakfast pictured above features two crisp waffles topped with Peach-Berry Sauce. Two slices of Canadian-style bacon count as Medium-Fat Meat Exchanges. The extra Fat Exchange that makes this breakfast possible is borrowed from dinner Exchanges. When lunch arrives, you'll find Seafaring Salmon Salad and piping-hot tomato soup are a satisfying combination. Exchange information for the tomato soup is included in the Exchange List for Packaged Foods on pages 31-35. Crackers or any other Bread Exchange can be substituted for the toasted rye bread. If soup and salad are all you need at lunch, you can save the pear halves and cream cheese for a snack later in the day. Dinner consists of Barbecued Ham Slice, fresh corn, Calorie Counter's Coleslaw, and watermelon.

breakfast ●●

DAILY MEAL PLAN		MENU A	
●●	2 Lean Meat Exchanges	●●●	2 1-oz. slices cooked Canadian-style bacon
●●	2 Bread Exchanges	●●●●	2 5-inch waffles
●	1 Fruit Exchange	●	Peach-Berry Sauce*
◖	½ Milk Exchange	◖	½ cup skim milk
●●	2 Fat Exchanges	●	tea with lemon
●	Free Exchanges		
			Extra Exchanges used:
		●	1 Fat Exchange

lunch

●●	2 Lean Meat Exchanges	●●●●	Seafaring Salmon Salad*
●●	2 Bread Exchanges	●	1 slice rye bread, toasted
●	1 Fruit Exchange	◖	1½ tsp. diet imitation margarine
●●	2 Vegetable Exchanges	●●	10 oz. prepared condensed tomato soup
●	1 Milk Exchange	●	1 small pear, halved
●●	2 Fat Exchanges	●	1 tbsp. cream cheese
●	Free Exchanges	●	1 cup skim milk
		●	coffee or tea

dinner

●●●●	4 Lean Meat Exchanges	●●●●	Barbecued Ham Slice*
		●	
●	1 Bread Exchange	●	1 small ear of corn
●	1 Fruit Exchange	●	1 tbsp. diet imitation margarine
●●	2 Vegetable Exchanges	●●	Calorie Counter's Coleslaw*
◖	½ Milk Exchange	●	1 cup watermelon balls
●●●	3 Fat Exchanges	◖	½ cup skim milk
●	Free Exchanges	●	coffee or tea
			Exchanges not used:
		●	1 Fat Exchange

breakfast

DAILY MEAL PLAN	MENU B
●● 2 Lean Meat Exchanges	●● 2 pork breakfast strips
●● 2 Bread Exchanges	2 slices French toast:
● 1 Fruit Exchange	●◖ 1 egg
◖ ½ Milk Exchange	●● 2 slices white bread
●● 2 Fat Exchanges	◖ 1½ tsp. diet imitation
● Free Exchanges	margarine
	● ½ cup fresh blueberries
	◖ ½ cup skim milk

lunch

DAILY MEAL PLAN	MENU B
●● 2 Lean Meat Exchanges	●●●◖ Fruity Ham Sandwiches*
	●●●
●● 2 Bread Exchanges	● Asparagus Bisque*
● 1 Fruit Exchange	◖ 3 saltine crackers
●● 2 Vegetable Exchanges	● ½ cup vegetable relishes
● 1 Milk Exchange	● 1 cup skim milk
●● 2 Fat Exchanges	
● Free Exchanges	

dinner

DAILY MEAL PLAN	MENU B
●●●● 4 Lean Meat Exchanges	●●● Spicy Marinated Pork Chops*
	◖● ●◖
● 1 Bread Exchange	● 1 slice Italian bread
● 1 Fruit Exchange	◖ 1½ tsp. diet imitation
●● 2 Vegetable Exchanges	margarine
◖ ½ Milk Exchange	● ⅛ avocado, sliced and
●●● 3 Fat Exchanges	served on a
● Free Exchanges	● lettuce-lined plate
	◖ Tangy Tomato Dressing*
	●● Orange Soufflé*
	◖ ½ cup skim milk

MENU C

- ½ cup cooked oatmeal
- ½ cup skim milk
- 2 tbsp. raisins
- 1 slice bread, toasted
- 1 tbsp. diet imitation margarine
- coffee or tea

Exchanges not used:

- 2 Lean Meat Exchanges
- 1 Fat Exchange

Onion Soup Gratiné*
Chef's Salad Bowl*

- 2 refrigerated buttermilk biscuits
- 1 tbsp. diet imitation margarine
- ¾ cup fresh strawberries
- 1 cup skim milk
- coffee or tea

Extra Exchanges used:

- 2 Lean Meat Exchanges

Cheese and Carrot Balls*
French Herbed Chicken*

Bean-Stuffed Tomatoes*

- 12 red grapes
- 3 tbsp. dairy sour cream
- Mint Chocolate Cream Puffs*
- coffee or tea

Extra Exchanges used:

- 1 Fat Exchange

menu planning tips

Wake up to a breakfast of pork breakfast strips, French toast, and blueberries on Menu B. Pork breakfast strips can be found on the Exchange List for Packaged Foods on pages 31-35. Two slices of pork breakfast strips supply only one Fat Exchange and one Lean Meat Exchange. Follow the list of Exchanges through the day and you will sample Fruity Ham Sandwiches, vegetable relishes, and Asparagus Bisque for lunch, and Spicy Marinated Pork Chops, Italian bread, avocado salad, and Orange Soufflé for dinner. If you prefer, save the vegetable relishes (your choice of any of the crispy Vegetable Exchanges served raw) for a mid-afternoon snack.

Menu C offers a hearty breakfast with a savings of two Lean Meat Exchanges and one Fat Exchange. Top the oatmeal with skim milk, add naturally sweet raisins, and you won't miss the sugar. Feast on Onion Soup Gratiné and Chef's Salad Bowl at noon. Tender biscuits can be topped with one tablespoon diet imitation margarine, but if you're yearning for butter, substitute one teaspoon for the Fat Exchange. Begin dinner with an appetizer of two Cheese and Carrot Balls. Bean-Stuffed Tomatoes complement savory French Herbed Chicken. A cluster of red grapes topped with a dab of sour cream provides a delicious garnish. Mint Chocolate Cream Puffs are the grand finale.

*see recipe section

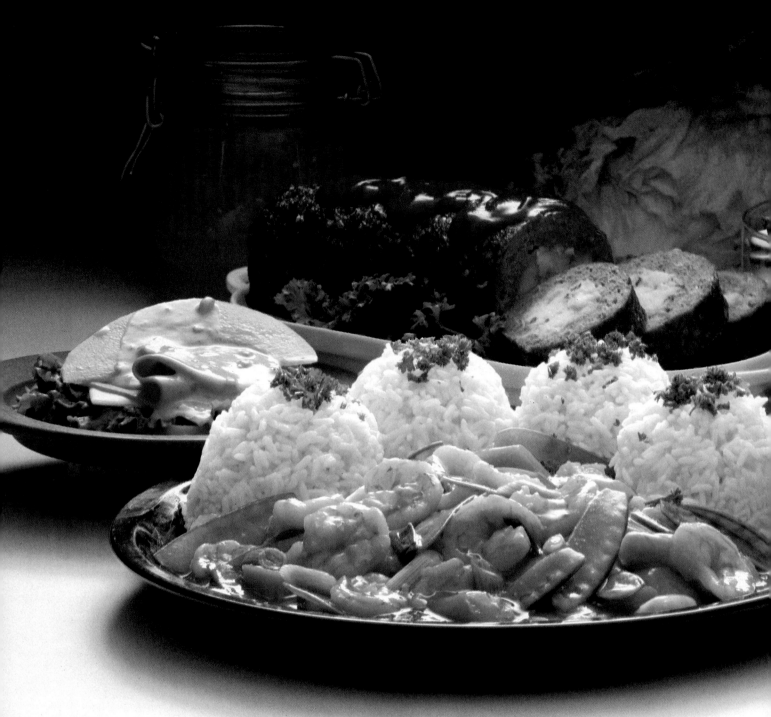

cooking with food exchanges

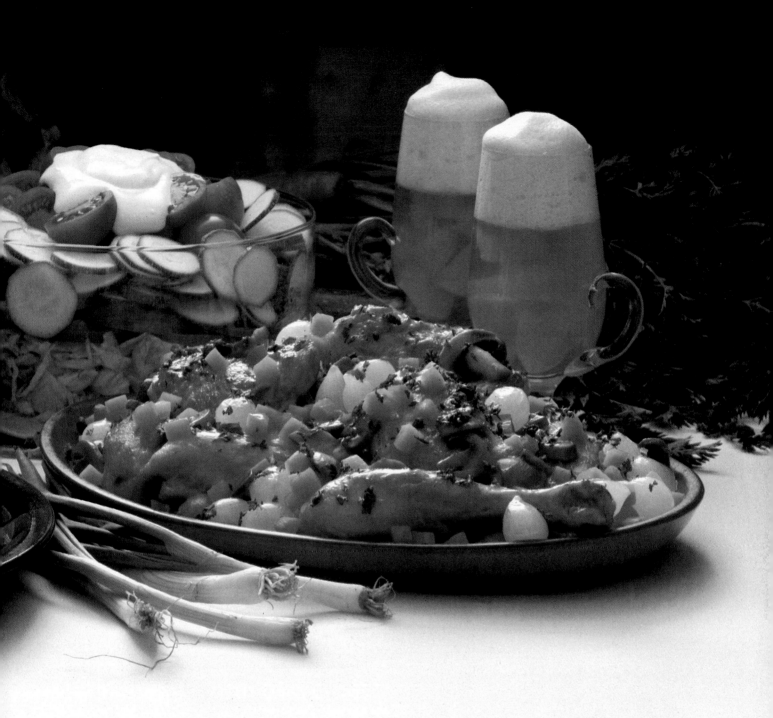

Discover how easy it is to cook dishes that are easy on the waistline with the Food Exchanges to guide you. The recipes in this chapter—all rated for Food Exchange values—demonstrate that eating doesn't have to be a bore when you diet. The Food Exchange reducing plan lets you savor a variety of flavor combinations that make you forget you're dieting. Recipes include (clockwise from back) Fruity Ham Sandwiches (see recipe, page 69); Meat and Potato Loaf (see recipe, page 59); Layered Vegetable Salad (see recipe, page 72); Layered Peach Dessert (see recipe, page 81); French Herbed Chicken (see recipe, page 63); and Polynesian Shrimp (see recipe, page 66).

beverages, appetizers, and soups

Strawberry Romanoff Swizzle

2 cups orange juice
2 cups frozen whole unsweetened
   strawberries, partially thawed
2 12-ounce cans low-calorie strawberry
   carbonated beverage, chilled
1 12-ounce can low-calorie lemon-lime
   carbonated beverage, chilled

In blender container combine orange juice and
berries. Cover; blend till pureed. Strain into large
pitcher. Pour carbonated beverages down side of
pitcher. Stir gently. Serve over ice in tall glasses. If
desired, garnish with fresh strawberries. Makes 8
servings. One serving (7.5 ounces) equals:

   ● 1 Fruit Exchange

Mexican-Style Hot Chocolate
pictured on the cover

3 tablespoons unsweetened cocoa powder
   Non-caloric liquid sweetener equal to 3
      tablespoons sugar
3½ inches stick cinnamon
3 cups skim milk
¼ teaspoon vanilla

Combine cocoa, non-caloric sweetener, stick cinnamon, and ⅔ cup *water*. Bring to boil, stirring
constantly; boil 1 minute longer. Stir in skim milk.
Cook till heated through *(do not boil)*. Add vanilla;
remove stick cinnamon. Beat with rotary beater. If
desired, garnish with additional cinnamon sticks.
Makes 4 servings. One serving (6 ounces) equals:

   ● 1 Milk Exchange

Citrus Frost

1½ cups orange sherbet
1 6-ounce can frozen tangerine juice
   concentrate
4 ice cubes
3 12-ounce cans low-calorie grapefruit
   carbonated beverage, chilled

In blender container combine orange sherbet,
tangerine juice concentrate, ice cubes, and 1 cup
cold *water*. Cover; blend till smooth. Pour into 6 tall
glasses. Pour carbonated beverage down sides of
glasses. Stir gently. Makes 6 servings. One serving
(10 ounces) equals:

   ● 1 Bread Exchange
   ○ 1 Fruit Exchange

Icy Tomato Tune-Up

2½ cups tomato juice
2 tablespoons lemon juice
1 teaspoon worcestershire sauce
⅛ teaspoon celery salt
5 drops bottled hot pepper sauce

Combine all ingredients. Chill well and serve *or*
pour into 8x8x2-inch baking dish and freeze about
1¼ hours or till slushy. Spoon into glasses. Makes 5
servings. One serving (4 ounces) equals:

   ● 1 Vegetable Exchange

*Citrus Frost, top left; Strawberry Romanoff Swizzle, top
middle; Asparagus Bisque, top right (see recipe, page
55); and Dilled Garden Dip, bottom (see recipe, page 54).*

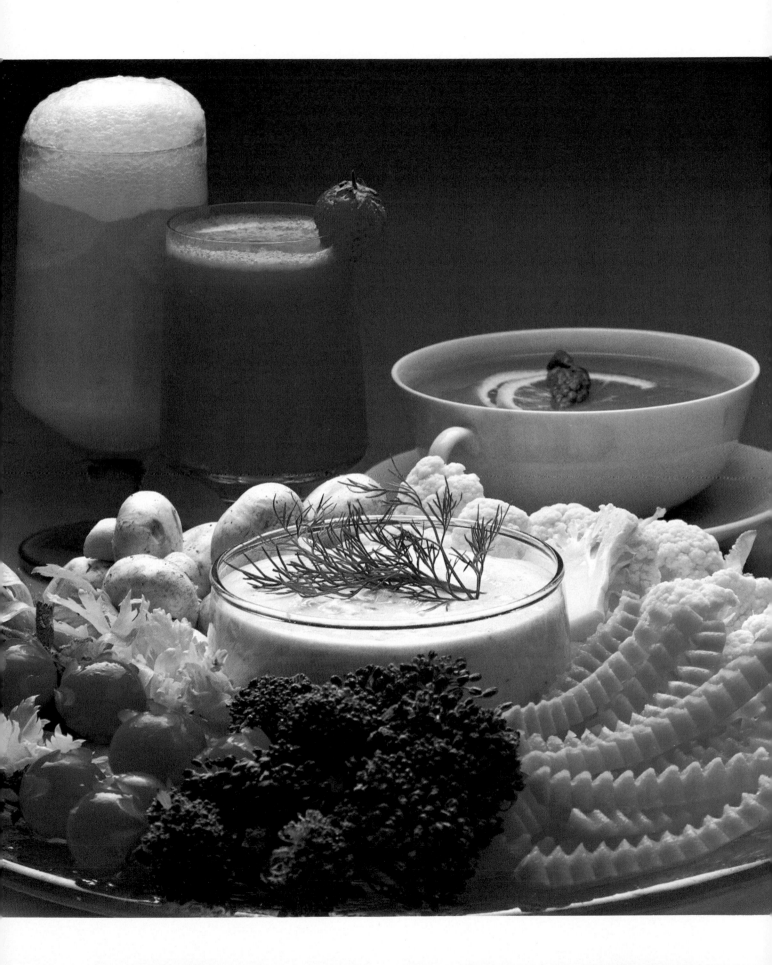

Herbed Mushrooms

  ⅔ cup dry red wine
  1 small onion, sliced and separated into rings
  ½ teaspoon dried basil, crushed
  ¼ teaspoon salt
  ⅛ teaspoon freshly ground pepper
  3 4-ounce cans whole mushrooms, drained
      Lettuce leaves
  2 tablespoons snipped parsley

In small saucepan combine wine, onion, basil, salt, and pepper. Bring to boil; add mushrooms. Cook over medium heat for 15 minutes or till most of the liquid evaporates. Pour into bowl; cover and chill. At serving time, drain and serve mushrooms on lettuce-lined plate. Sprinkle with parsley. Makes 8 servings. One serving (¼ cup) equals:

  ◖ ½ Vegetable Exchange

Olive Meatballs

  1 beaten egg
  ½ cup soft bread crumbs (⅔ slice bread)
  ⅓ cup pizza sauce
  ¼ cup finely chopped onion
  1 pound ground beef (15% fat)
  36 medium pimiento-stuffed green olives, drained

In medium bowl combine egg, bread crumbs, pizza sauce, onion, ½ teaspoon *salt,* and dash *pepper.* Add ground beef; mix well. Shape about *1 tablespoon* of meat mixture evenly around each olive to form round meatballs. Place in 13x9x2-inch baking dish. Bake in 375° oven about 20 minutes. Serve warm on wooden picks. Makes 18 servings. One serving (2 meatballs) equals:

  ● 1 Lean Meat Exchange

  ◖ ½ Fat Exchange

Cheese and Carrot Balls

  3 ounces neufchatel cheese, softened
  ½ cup shredded low-calorie process cheese product (2 ounces)
  1 cup finely shredded carrot
  ⅓ cup grape nuts cereal
  2 tablespoons finely snipped parsley

In small bowl beat neufchatel cheese and process cheese. Pat shredded carrot dry with paper toweling. Stir shredded carrot into cheese mixture. Cover; chill at least 1 hour. Combine cereal and parsley; set aside. Shape cheese-carrot mixture into sixteen 1-inch balls. Roll balls in cereal-parsley mixture, pressing into cheese-carrot balls to coat. Cover; chill up to 1 hour. Makes 8 servings. One serving (2 cheese and carrot balls) equals:

  ◖ ½ Lean Meat Exchange

  ◖ ½ Bread Exchange

Dilled Garden Dip
pictured on page 53

  2 cups lowfat cottage cheese (no more than 2% butterfat)
  2 tablespoons tarragon vinegar
  1 tablespoon finely chopped green onion
  1 tablespoon snipped parsley
  1 teaspoon snipped fresh mint
  ½ teaspoon dried dillweed
      Dash freshly ground pepper
  4 cups fresh vegetable dippers (broccoli, carrots, cauliflower, celery, cucumber, mushrooms, cherry tomatoes, zucchini, green onion, and green pepper)
      Radishes

In blender container combine cottage cheese and vinegar. Cover; blend till smooth. Stir in onion, parsley, mint, dried dillweed, and pepper. Cover and chill thoroughly. If desired, garnish with fresh dillweed. Serve dip with vegetable dippers and radishes. Makes 8 servings. One serving (¼ cup dip and ½ cup vegetables except radishes, which can be eaten in any amount) equals:

  ● 1 Lean Meat Exchange

  ◗ 1 Vegetable Exchange

Asparagus Bisque

pictured on page 53

2 10-ounce packages frozen cut asparagus
3½ cups water
1 medium onion, quartered
2 tablespoons lemon juice
4 teaspoons instant chicken bouillon
granules
1 to 2 teaspoons curry powder
Dash pepper

In large saucepan combine asparagus, water, onion, lemon juice, bouillon granules, curry powder, and pepper. Bring to boil; simmer, covered, 8 to 12 minutes or till asparagus is just tender. Place *half* the asparagus mixture in blender container. Cover; blend till smooth. Pour into bowl. Repeat with remaining asparagus mixture. Serve hot or cover and chill at least 4 hours. If desired, garnish each serving with a lemon slice and an asparagus tip. Makes 6 servings. One serving (1 cup) equals:

● 1 Vegetable Exchange

Herbed Tomato Soup

pictured on the cover

2½ cups tomato juice
1 10½-ounce can *condensed* beef broth
1 tablespoon lemon juice
1 teaspoon worcestershire sauce
¼ teaspoon dried basil, crushed
¼ teaspoon dried thyme, crushed
6 thin lemon slices *or* snipped parsley

In medium saucepan combine tomato juice, beef broth, lemon juice, worcestershire sauce, basil, and thyme. Bring to boil; simmer, covered, 5 minutes. Ladle into bowls. Garnish each serving with a thin lemon slice or snipped parsley. Makes 6 servings. One serving (⅔ cup) equals:

● 1 Vegetable Exchange

Cucumber-Buttermilk Soup

1 quart buttermilk, made from skim milk (no
more than 0.5% butterfat)
2 cucumbers, peeled, seeded, and shredded
(1 cup)
2 tablespoons snipped parsley
1 tablespoon sliced green onion
1 teaspoon salt
Dash pepper

In large bowl combine buttermilk, shredded cucumber, parsley, onion, salt, and pepper. Cover and chill till serving time. Makes 5 servings. One serving (1 cup) equals:

● 1 Milk Exchange

Onion Soup Gratiné

1 large onion, thinly sliced (1 cup)
1 tablespoon diet imitation margarine
2 10½-ounce cans *condensed* beef broth
1½ cups water
1 to 2 tablespoons dry sherry
½ teaspoon worcestershire sauce
Dash pepper
6 melba toast rounds
6 tablespoons grated parmesan cheese

In large saucepan cook onion in margarine, covered, over low heat about 20 minutes or till lightly browned, stirring occasionally. Add beef broth, water, sherry, and worcestershire sauce. Bring to boil; season with pepper. Pour into oven-proof cups or small bowls. Float melba toast on top of onion soup; sprinkle each toast piece with *1 tablespoon* of the parmesan cheese. Broil 3 to 4 inches from heat about 2 minutes or till browned. Makes 6 servings. One serving (¾ cup) equals:

● 1 Lean Meat Exchange

◖ ½ Bread Exchange

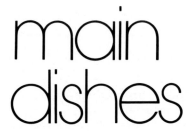

main dishes

Stir-Fried Beef and Spinach

1¼ **pounds boneless beef round steak, fat trimmed**
2 **tablespoons soy sauce**
¼ **teaspoon Five Spice Powder**
¼ **cup water**
2 **teaspoons cornstarch**
¼ **teaspoon instant beef bouillon granules**
1 **tablespoon cooking oil**
1 **teaspoon grated gingerroot**
8 **ounces small fresh spinach leaves (6 cups)**
½ **cup sliced water chestnuts**

Partially freeze beef; slice thinly into bite-size strips. Combine beef, soy sauce, and Five Spice Powder; let stand at room temperature 15 minutes. In small bowl blend water into cornstarch; add bouillon granules and set aside. Preheat wok or large skillet over high heat; add oil. Stir-fry gingerroot in hot oil 30 seconds. Add *half* the beef to hot wok; stir-fry 2 to 3 minutes or till browned. Remove beef. Stir-fry remaining beef 2 to 3 minutes. Return all beef to wok. Stir cornstarch mixture; stir into beef. Cook and stir till thickened and bubbly. Stir in spinach and water chestnuts; cook, covered, 1 to 2 minutes. Serve at once. Makes 6 servings.

Five Spice Powder: In small bowl combine 1 teaspoon ground *cinnamon;* 1 teaspoon crushed *aniseed or* 1 star *anise,* ground; ¼ teaspoon crushed *fennel seed;* ¼ teaspoon freshly ground *pepper or* ¼ teaspoon crushed *Szechwan pepper;* and ⅛ teaspoon ground *cloves.* Store in covered container. (Or, purchase five spice powder at Oriental food stores.)
One serving (⅔ cup) equals:

● ● ● ◖ 3½ Lean Meat Exchanges

● 1 Vegetable Exchange

◖ ½ Fat Exchange

Beef Burgundy

¾ **pound boneless beef sirloin steak, fat trimmed**
4 **teaspoons cooking oil**
4 **teaspoons cornstarch**
1 **medium onion, sliced and separated into rings**
½ **cup burgundy**
½ **cup water**
1 **teaspoon instant chicken bouillon granules**
⅛ **teaspoon dried oregano, crushed**
⅛ **teaspoon dried thyme, crushed**
1 **bay leaf**
Dash pepper
1 **cup sliced fresh mushrooms**
2 **cups hot cooked rice**

Partially freeze beef; slice thinly into bite-size strips. In 2-quart saucepan cook *half* the beef in *half* the hot oil over medium-high heat till browned. Remove beef. Repeat with remaining beef and oil. Return all beef to pan. Stir in cornstarch. Add onion, burgundy, water, bouillon granules, oregano, thyme, bay leaf, and pepper. Cook, covered, over low heat 35 to 45 minutes or till tender, adding mushrooms 5 minutes before end of cooking time. Remove bay leaf. Serve beef mixture over hot cooked rice. Makes 4 servings. One serving (about ½ cup beef mixture and ½ cup cooked rice) equals:

● ● ● 3 Lean Meat Exchanges

● 1 Bread Exchange

● 1 Vegetable Exchange

● 1 Fat Exchange

New England Boiled Dinner, top (see recipe, page 58); Stir-Fried Beef and Spinach, center left; and Skillet Spaghetti, bottom right (see recipe, page 58).

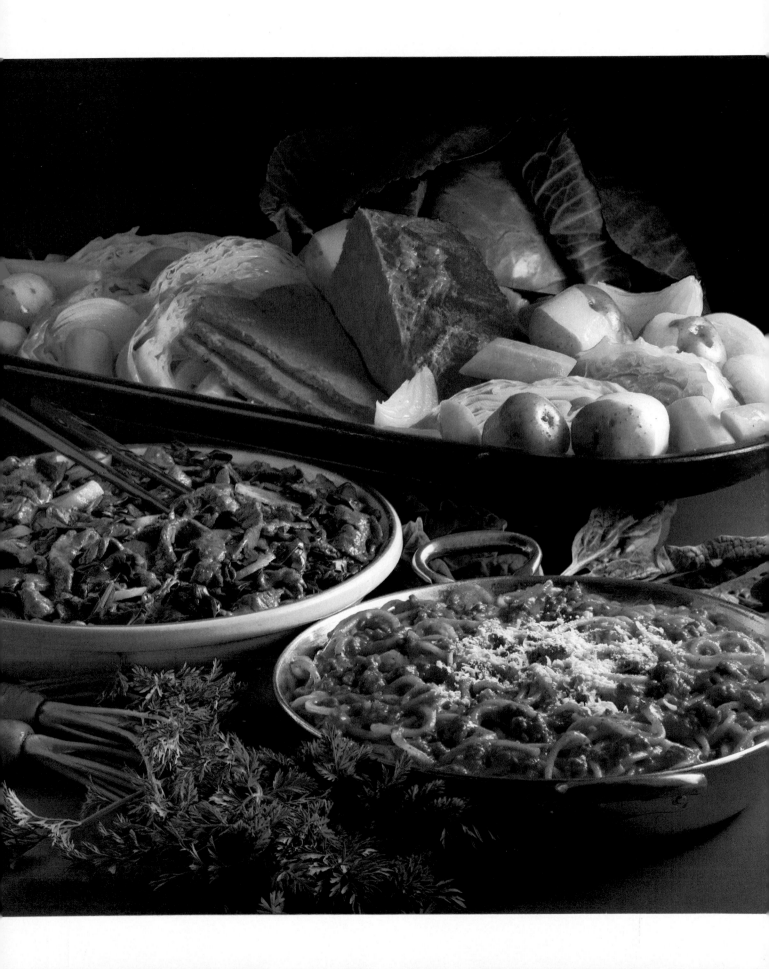

New England Boiled Dinner
pictured on page 57

1 3-pound corned beef round, fat trimmed
2 cloves garlic, minced
2 bay leaves
8 tiny new potatoes
4 medium carrots, quartered
2 small onions, quartered
1 medium head cabbage, cut into 8 wedges

In Dutch oven cover corned beef with *water*. Add garlic and bay leaves. Bring to boil; simmer, covered, 2½ hours. Remove meat. Add potatoes, carrots, and onions. Cook, covered, 10 minutes; add cabbage. Cook, covered, 15 to 20 minutes. Add meat; heat through. Drain meat and vegetables; season to taste. Serves 8. One serving equals:

● ● ● ◖ 3½ Lean Meat Exchanges

◖ ½ Bread Exchange

● ● 2 Vegetable Exchanges

Old Fashioned Beef Stew

1¼ pounds boneless beef round steak, cut into
    1-inch cubes and fat trimmed
1 tablespoon diet imitation margarine
1 teaspoon worcestershire sauce
2 bay leaves
1 clove garlic, minced
½ teaspoon paprika
    Dash ground cloves
8 medium carrots, quartered
4 small potatoes, peeled and quartered
4 small onions, quartered
1 tablespoon cornstarch

In Dutch oven brown beef in margarine. Add next 5 ingredients, 1½ cups hot *water*, 1½ teaspoons *salt*, and ¼ teaspoon *pepper*. Cook, covered, 1¼ hours; stir often. Remove bay leaves; add vegetables. Cook, covered, 30 to 45 minutes. Drain; reserve liquid. Skim fat. Add water to liquid to equal 1¼ cups; return to Dutch oven. Combine cornstarch and ¼ cup cold *water;* stir into hot liquid. Cook and stir till thickened; stir in beef and vegetables. Heat through. Serves 8. One serving (1 cup) equals:

● ● ◖ 2½ Lean Meat Exchanges

● 1 Bread Exchange

● 1 Vegetable Exchange

Skillet Spaghetti
pictured on page 57

1 pound ground beef (15% fat)
1 18-ounce can tomato juice
1 6-ounce can tomato paste
2 tablespoons minced dried onion
1½ teaspoons chili powder
1 teaspoon garlic salt
1 teaspoon dried oregano, crushed
1 7-ounce package spaghetti
7 tablespoons grated parmesan cheese

Combine first 7 ingredients, 3 cups *water,* and 1 teaspoon *salt*. Bring to boil. Simmer, covered, 30 minutes; stir often. Add spaghetti; simmer, covered, 30 minutes. Stir often. Serve with cheese. Makes 7 servings. One serving (1 cup) equals:

● ● ◖ 2½ Lean Meat Exchanges

● ◖ 1½ Bread Exchanges

● ◖ 1½ Vegetable Exchanges

● ◖ 1½ Fat Exchanges

No Crust Pizza

1 2-ounce can chopped mushrooms
1 slightly beaten egg
1 cup soft bread crumbs (1¼ slices bread)
½ teaspoon dried oregano, crushed
1 pound ground beef (15% fat)
2 1-ounce slices mozzarella cheese
½ of an 8-ounce can (½ cup) pizza sauce
¼ cup chopped onion
2 tablespoons chopped green pepper

Drain mushrooms; reserve liquid. Add *water* to equal ⅓ cup liquid. Combine the liquid, egg, crumbs, oregano, ½ teaspoon *salt,* and dash *pepper;* let stand 5 minutes. Add beef; mix well. Pat beef mixture into 9-inch pie plate to form crust. Cut cheese into 8 triangles; layer *half* atop beef mixture. Top with pizza sauce, mushrooms, onion, and green pepper. Bake in 350° oven 45 minutes. Top with remaining cheese; bake 5 minutes. Remove to serving platter, using two spatulas. Makes 8 servings. One serving (⅛ pizza) equals:

● ● ◖ 2½ Lean Meat Exchanges

● 1 Vegetable Exchange

● 1 Fat Exchange

Meat and Potato Loaf
pictured on page 50

2 medium potatoes, peeled and cut up
1 tablespoon snipped parsley
⅛ teaspoon dried thyme, crushed
⅛ teaspoon dried marjoram, crushed
  Salt
  Pepper
2 beaten eggs
½ cup finely crushed saltine crackers
    (14 crackers)
⅓ cup tomato sauce
¼ cup finely chopped onion
2 tablespoons finely chopped green pepper
¾ teaspoon salt
1½ pounds ground beef (15% fat)
¼ cup catsup
¼ teaspoon dry mustard

Cook potatoes, covered, in boiling salted water about 20 minutes or till tender; drain, reserving liquid. Mash potatoes, adding about 3 *tablespoons* of the reserved liquid to make stiff consistency. Stir in parsley, thyme, and marjoram. Season to taste with salt and pepper; set aside.

In large bowl stir together eggs, cracker crumbs, tomato sauce, onion, green pepper, and ¾ teaspoon salt. Add beef; mix well. On waxed paper pat beef mixture to a 10x8-inch rectangle; spoon potato mixture lengthwise down center of beef mixture. Fold sides over potato mixture; seal. Place loaf, seam side down, on 15x10½x2-inch baking pan. Remove paper. Bake in 350° oven 45 minutes or till done. Heat together catsup and mustard; spoon over meat loaf. If desired, garnish with fresh parsley. Makes 8 servings. One serving (⅛ meat loaf) equals:

● ● ● 3 Lean Meat Exchanges
(½ Bread Exchange
● 1 Vegetable Exchange
●(1½ Fat Exchanges

Taco Compuesto
pictured on the cover

1 pound ground beef (15% fat)
½ cup chopped onion
2 tablespoons chopped canned green chili peppers
1 clove garlic, minced
1 teaspoon chili powder
1½ cups chopped tomato
3 tablespoons low-calorie Italian salad dressing (no more than 8 calories per tablespoon)
½ teaspoon seasoned salt
8 taco shells
1 cup shredded lettuce
½ cup shredded low-calorie process cheese product (2 ounces)
½ cup taco sauce

Cook beef, onion, chili peppers, and garlic till beef is browned; drain. Stir in chili powder and ½ teaspoon *salt*. Combine tomato, salad dressing, and seasoned salt. Spoon beef mixture into taco shells; top with tomato mixture, lettuce, and cheese. Pass taco sauce. Makes 4 servings. One serving (2 tacos and 2 tablespoons taco sauce) equals:

● ● ● (3½ Lean Meat Exchanges
● ● 2 Bread Exchanges
● ● 2 Vegetable Exchanges
●(1½ Fat Exchanges

Barbecued Ham Slice

½ cup catsup
2 tablespoons finely chopped onion
1 tablespoon worcestershire sauce
2 teaspoons lemon juice
2 teaspoons prepared mustard
¼ teaspoon chili powder
1 1½-pound fully cooked ham slice, cut 1 inch thick and fat trimmed

For sauce, combine all ingredients *except* ham. Bring to boil. Slash edges of ham; brush with some sauce. Place ham on unheated rack in broiler pan. Broil 3 to 4 inches from heat 5 to 6 minutes on each side, brushing with sauce once. Makes 6 servings. One serving (4 ounces) equals:

● ● ● ● 4 Lean Meat Exchanges

● 1 Vegetable Exchange

Spicy Marinated Pork Chops

1 cup vegetable juice cocktail
3 tablespoons finely chopped onion
3 tablespoons finely chopped green pepper
3 tablespoons lemon juice
2 tablespoons low-calorie Italian salad dressing mix
2 tablespoons worcestershire sauce
Few drops bottled hot pepper sauce
4 pork loin chops, cut ½ inch thick and fat trimmed

For marinade, in plastic bag combine all ingredients *except* chops; add chops. Close bag securely; place in an 8x8x2-inch baking dish. Refrigerate 8 hours or overnight. Drain; reserve marinade. Place chops on unheated rack in broiler pan. Broil chops 3 to 4 inches from heat 6 minutes on each side or till done. Heat marinade and serve with chops. Makes 4 servings. One serving (1 chop and ¼ cup marinade) equals:

● ● ● 3 Lean Meat Exchanges

● ◖ 1½ Vegetable Exchanges

● ◖ 1½ Fat Exchanges

Pineapple and Pork Stir-Fry

12 ounces pork tenderloin *or* boneless pork, fat trimmed
1 small fresh pineapple
½ cup orange juice
¼ cup soy sauce
½ teaspoon instant chicken bouillon granules
1 clove garlic, minced
⅛ teaspoon pepper
2 tablespoons cold water
4 teaspoons cornstarch
1 medium red *or* green pepper, cut in 1-inch squares
1 tablespoon cooking oil

Partially freeze pork; slice thinly into bite-size strips. Set aside. Remove pineapple crown. Cut off peel; remove all eyes from fruit by cutting diagonal wedge-shaped grooves in the pineapple. Cut pineapple lengthwise into 8 wedges, reserving any juice. Cut off center core from each wedge. In small bowl combine reserved pineapple juice, orange juice, soy sauce, bouillon granules, garlic, and pepper; set aside. In small bowl blend cold water into cornstarch; set aside.

In wok or large skillet stir-fry pork and red or green pepper in hot oil over high heat 3 to 4 minutes or till pork is just browned. Remove from wok. Pour juice mixture into wok; add pineapple wedges. Cook, covered, 2 minutes. Remove wedges with slotted spoon and arrange on platter; keep warm. Return pork and peppers to hot liquid in wok. Stir cornstarch mixture; add to wok. Cook and stir till thickened and bubbly. (If sauce is thick, add a few tablespoons water.) Spoon pork mixture atop pineapple wedges. Makes 4 servings. One serving (½ cup pork mixture and 2 wedges pineapple) equals:

● ● ● 3 Lean Meat Exchanges

○ ○ 2 Fruit Exchanges

◖ ½ Vegetable Exchange

● ● 2 Fat Exchanges

Veal and Peppers Italiano, top (see recipe, page 62); Barbecued Ham Slice, center; and Athenian Lamb Kabobs, bottom (see recipe, page 62).

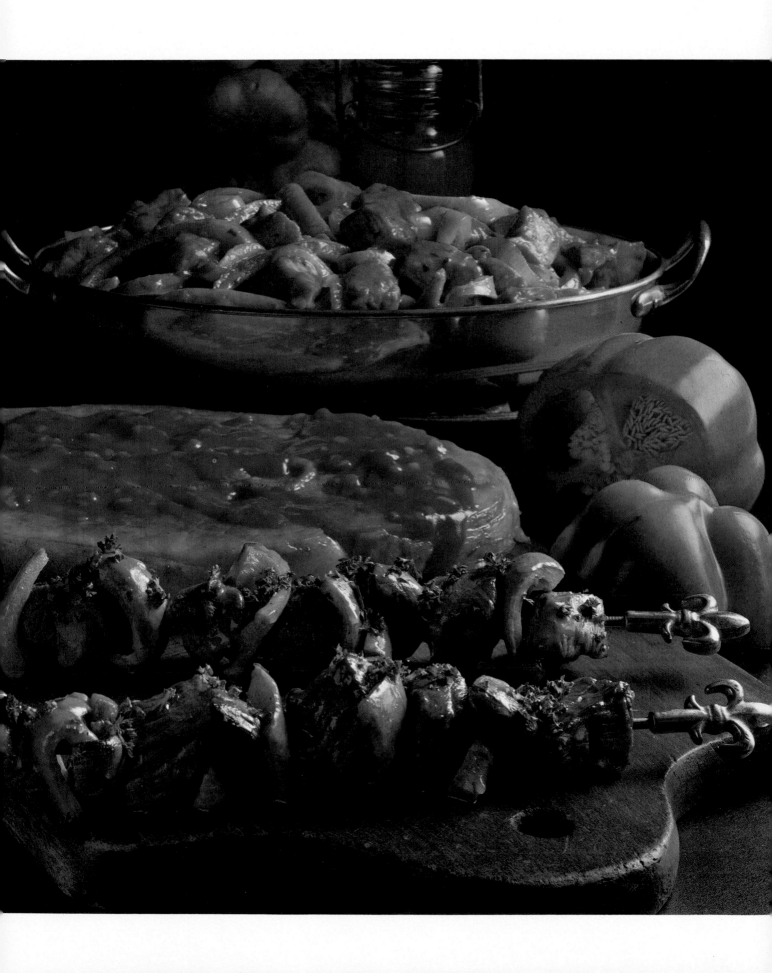

Fruited Lamb Chops
pictured on page 38

    1 16-ounce can peach slices (juice pack)
    2 teaspoons cornstarch
    ½ teaspoon ground ginger
    ¼ teaspoon ground nutmeg
    2 tablespoons diet imitation margarine
    1 tablespoon lemon juice
    1 teaspoon soy sauce
    8 lamb loin chops, cut ¾ inch thick

Drain peaches, reserving juice; halve peaches lengthwise. Combine cornstarch and spices; blend in juice. Cook and stir till thickened; stir in margarine, lemon juice, and soy sauce. Trim fat from chops; brush chops with some sauce. Broil 3 to 4 inches from heat 9 to 10 minutes, turning and brushing with sauce once. Stir peaches into remaining sauce; heat through; serve with chops. Serves 8. One serving (1 chop and ¼ cup sauce) equals:

    ●● 2 Lean Meat Exchanges
     ◖ ½ Fruit Exchange
     ◖ ½ Fat Exchange

Veal and Peppers Italiano
Pictured on page 61

    1 pound boneless lean veal
    1 tablespoon diet imitation margarine
    1 10½-ounce can tomato puree
    1 cup chicken broth
    1 clove garlic, minced
    ½ teaspoon dried basil, crushed
    ½ teaspoon dried oregano, crushed
    2 medium green peppers, cut into strips
    1 medium onion, sliced
    2 cups hot cooked rice

Cut veal into 1-inch cubes; trim fat. Brown veal in margarine. Stir in next 5 ingredients, ¾ teaspoon *salt,* and ⅛ teaspoon *pepper.* Simmer, covered, 25 minutes. Add green peppers and onion; cook, covered, 20 minutes. Serve with rice. Makes 4 servings. One serving (1 cup veal mixture and ½ cup rice) equals:

    ●●●● 4 Lean Meat Exchanges
       ● 1 Bread Exchange
      ●● 2 Vegetable Exchanges
       ◖ ½ Fat Exchange

Athenian Lamb Kabobs
pictured on page 61

    ¾ cup low-calorie French salad dressing (no
         more than 25 calories per tablespoon)
    3 tablespoons lime juice
    ½ teaspoon dried oregano, crushed
    ¼ teaspoon dried tarragon, crushed
    1½ pounds boneless lean lamb, fat trimmed
    2 cups small fresh mushrooms
    2 medium green peppers

For marinade, combine salad dressing, lime juice, and herbs. Cut lamb into 1-inch cubes; add to marinade. Cover; let stand 2 hours at room temperature, stirring occasionally. Drain; reserve marinade. Sprinkle lamb with *salt.* Pour boiling *water* over mushrooms; let stand 1 minute and drain. Cut green peppers into 1-inch squares. Alternate lamb and vegetables on 6 skewers. Broil 4 inches from heat 10 to 12 minutes, turning and basting with marinade occasionally. If desired, sprinkle with snipped parsley. Makes 6 servings. One serving (1 kabob) equals:

    ●●● 3 Lean Meat Exchanges
      ● 1 Vegetable Exchange
      ● 1 Fat Exchange

Veal Scallopini

    12 ounces boneless veal leg round steak, cut
          ¼ inch thick and fat trimmed
     2 tablespoons diet imitation margarine
     ¼ cup dry sherry
     ¾ teaspoon instant chicken bouillon granules
     1 4-ounce can sliced mushrooms, drained
     2 tablespoons snipped parsley

Cut veal into 4 pieces; pound to ⅛-inch thickness. Cook veal in hot margarine 1 to 1½ minutes on each side. Remove; keep warm. For sauce, in same pan add sherry, bouillon granules, ½ cup *water,* and ⅛ teaspoon *pepper* to drippings. Boil sauce 3 to 4 minutes or till reduced to ⅓ cup. Stir in mushrooms and parsley. Heat through. Pour over veal. Makes 4 servings. One serving (1 piece veal and 3 tablespoons sauce) equals:

    ●●● 3 Lean Meat Exchanges
      ◖ ½ Fat Exchange

French Herbed Chicken
pictured on page 50

- 1 3-pound broiler-fryer chicken, cut up
- 1 tablespoon cooking oil
- 1 cup sauterne
- 1 8-ounce can (1 cup) stewed onions, drained
- 1 cup sliced fresh mushrooms
- ½ cup coarsely chopped carrot
- 2 to 3 stalks celery, cut up
- 2 tablespoons snipped parsley
- ¼ teaspoon dried thyme, crushed
- 1 clove garlic, minced
- 1 bay leaf

Remove wing tips and skin from chicken; brown chicken in hot oil. Drain. Season chicken to taste. Add remaining ingredients. Bring to boil; simmer, covered, 45 minutes. Remove celery and bay leaf; discard. Remove chicken and vegetables; keep warm. Boil sauce 5 minutes or till reduced to ½ cup. Makes 6 servings. One serving (⅙ recipe) equals

 3½ Lean Meat Exchanges

(½ Vegetable Exchange

(½ Fat Exchange

Spicy Baked Chicken

- ¼ cup all-purpose flour
- 2 tablespoons snipped parsley
- 1 tablespoon low-calorie Italian salad dressing mix
- 2 teaspoons diet imitation margarine
- ½ teaspoon paprika
- 3 tablespoons water
- 1 3-pound broiler-fryer chicken, cut up

In small bowl stir together flour, parsley, salad dressing mix, margarine, and paprika. Blend in water. Remove wing tips and skin from chicken. Spread flour mixture over skinned chicken pieces. Place chicken in ungreased 15x10x1-inch baking pan. Bake in 375° oven 50 to 60 minutes. *Do not turn.* Makes 4 servings. One serving (¼ recipe) equals:

 3½ Lean Meat Exchanges

(½ Bread Exchange

Cheese-Stuffed Chicken

- 2 8-ounce whole chicken breasts, skinned, split, and boned
- 4 3x1-inch slices monterey jack cheese
- 1 egg
- 2 teaspoons grated parmesan cheese
- 1 teaspoon snipped parsley
- ½ teaspoon instant chicken bouillon granules
- 2 tablespoons all-purpose flour
- 2 tablespoons cooking oil

In thickest side of each chicken piece, cut a pocket just large enough for cheese slice. Place a cheese slice in each pocket. Beat together egg, parmesan cheese, parsley, bouillon granules, and dash *pepper.* Coat chicken with flour and dip in egg mixture; brown in hot oil 2 to 3 minutes on each side. Transfer to 10x6x2-inch baking dish. Bake in 375° oven 8 to 10 minutes. Makes 4 servings. One serving (1 piece) equals:

● ● ● 3 Lean Meat Exchanges

● ● 2 Fat Exchanges

Teriyaki Chicken Kabobs

- ¼ cup soy sauce
- ¼ cup dry sherry
- ¼ cup water
- 1 clove garlic, minced
- 1 teaspoon grated gingerroot *or* ¼ teaspoon ground ginger
- 2 8-ounce whole chicken breasts, skinned, split, boned, and cut into 1-inch cubes
- 6 large green onions, bias-sliced into 1-inch lengths
- 4 cherry tomatoes

Combine soy sauce, sherry, water, garlic, and gingerroot or ginger. Boil 1 minute; cool. Marinate chicken and green onion in soy mixture 30 minutes at room temperature, stirring once to coat all pieces. Drain; reserve marinade. Alternate chicken and onion pieces on 4 skewers. Broil kabobs 4 inches from heat 4 to 5 minutes. Place a cherry tomato on end of each skewer. Turn; broil kabobs 4 to 5 minutes longer, brushing occasionally with marinade. Makes 4 servings. One serving (1 kabob) equals:

● ● 2 Lean Meat Exchanges

● 1 Vegetable Exchange

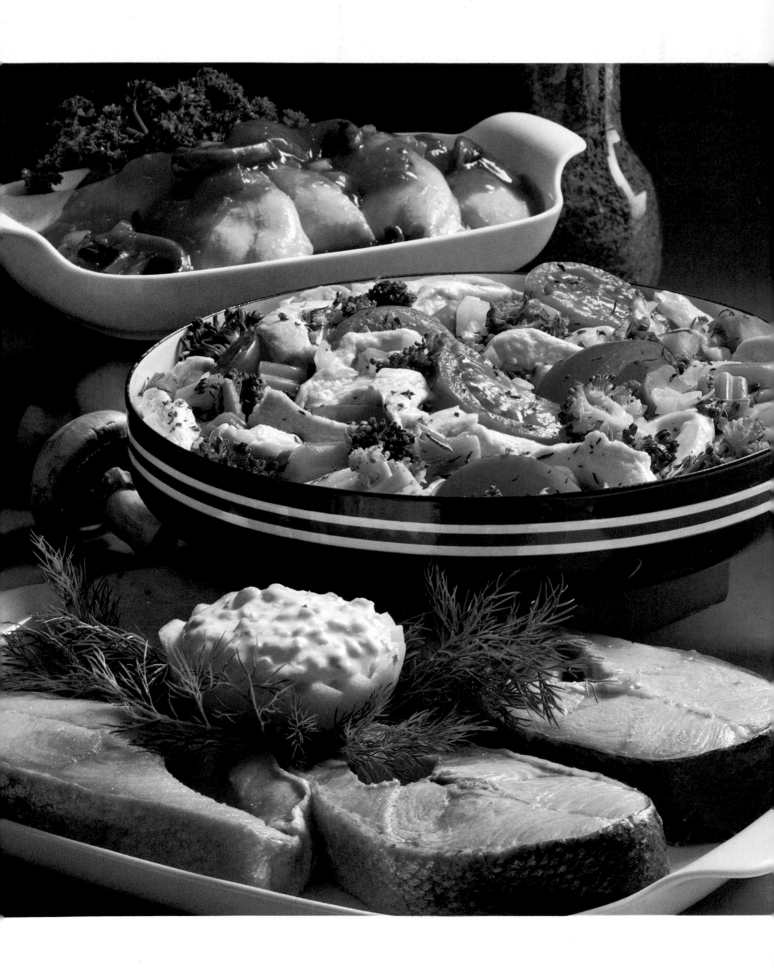

Chicken-Broccoli Skillet

1 10-ounce package frozen cut broccoli
2 8-ounce whole chicken breasts, skinned,
   split, boned, and cut into ½-inch-wide
   strips
¼ cup chopped onion
2 tablespoons diet imitation margarine
1 teaspoon lemon juice
¼ teaspoon dried thyme, crushed
3 medium tomatoes, cut in wedges

Thaw broccoli. Season chicken with salt and pepper. Cook chicken and onion quickly in hot margarine till just done. Stir in broccoli, lemon juice, thyme, ¾ teaspoon *salt*, and ⅛ teaspoon *pepper.* Cook, covered, 6 minutes. Add tomatoes. Cook, covered, 3 to 4 minutes. Makes 4 servings. One serving (1¼ cups) equals:

● ● ◖ 2½ Lean Meat Exchanges

● ● 2 Vegetable Exchanges

◖ ½ Fat Exchange

Turkey-Asparagus Pilaf

1 6¾-ounce package quick-cooking long
   grain and wild rice mix
1 10-ounce package frozen cut asparagus
3 cups cooked turkey cut into strips
⅓ cup chicken broth
¼ cup sliced almonds
2 tablespoons dry sherry
2 tablespoons white wine vinegar

Prepare rice mix according to package directions *except* substitute *diet imitation margarine* for the butter. Cook asparagus according to package directions; drain. Add asparagus, turkey, chicken broth, almonds, sherry, and vinegar to rice; heat through. Season to taste with *salt* and *pepper.* Makes 8 servings. One serving (1 cup) equals:

● ● 2 Lean Meat Exchanges

● 1 Bread Exchange

● 1 Vegetable Exchange

● 1 Fat Exchange

Chicken Cacciatore, top; Chicken-Broccoli Skillet, center; and Lemon Poached Salmon and Tartar Sauce, bottom (see recipes, page 66).

Chicken Cacciatore

½ of an 8-ounce can (½ cup) tomatoes
¾ cup sliced fresh mushrooms
¼ cup chopped onion
¼ cup chopped green pepper
3 tablespoons dry red wine
1 clove garlic, minced
½ teaspoon dried oregano, crushed
2 8-ounce whole chicken breasts, skinned,
   split, and boned
   Paprika
2 teaspoons cornstarch

In medium skillet cut up *undrained* tomatoes. Add next 6 ingredients, ½ teaspoon *salt,* and dash *pepper;* place chicken atop. Bring to boil; simmer, covered, 25 minutes. Remove chicken; sprinkle with paprika. Keep warm. Combine cornstarch and 2 tablespoons cold *water;* stir into skillet mixture. Cook and stir till thickened; cook 1 minute longer. Spoon sauce over chicken. If desired, garnish with a sprig of parsley. Makes 4 servings. One serving (½ breast and ⅓ cup sauce) equals:

● ● ◖ 2½ Lean Meat Exchanges

● 1 Vegetable Exchange

Polynesian Shrimp
pictured on page 50

12 ounces fresh *or* frozen shelled shrimp,
    halved lengthwise
1½ cups carrots bias-sliced into ½-inch lengths
 ⅔ cup cold water
  1 tablespoon cornstarch
 ½ of a 6-ounce can (6 tablespoons) frozen
    pineapple juice concentrate, thawed
  2 tablespoons soy sauce
  1 teaspoon instant chicken bouillon granules
  1 tablespoon cooking oil
  2 teaspoons grated gingerroot
  1 clove garlic, minced
  1 6-ounce package frozen pea pods, thawed
 ¼ cup green onion bias-sliced into ½-inch
    lengths
  2 cups hot cooked rice

Thaw shrimp, if frozen. In saucepan cook carrots in small amount of boiling salted water 5 to 7 minutes or till just tender; drain well. Blend ⅔ cup cold water into cornstarch; stir in pineapple juice, soy sauce, and chicken bouillon granules; set aside.

Preheat wok or large skillet over high heat; add oil. Stir-fry gingerroot and garlic in hot oil for 30 seconds. Add the carrots, pea pods, and green onion; stir-fry 1 minute or till heated through. Remove the vegetables.

Stir-fry the shrimp in hot oil 7 to 8 minutes or till shrimp are done. Push shrimp away from center of wok or skillet. Stir the soy mixture and add to center of wok or skillet. Cook and stir till thickened and bubbly. Stir in vegetables; cover and cook 1 minute. Serve shrimp mixture at once with hot cooked rice. If desired, sprinkle rice with parsley. Makes 4 servings. One serving (1 cup shrimp mixture and ½ cup rice) equals:

● ● ● 3 Lean Meat Exchanges

●   1 Bread Exchange

◖   1½ Fruit Exchanges

● ●   2 Vegetable Exchanges

●   1 Fat Exchange

Lemon Poached Salmon
pictured on page 64

4 6-ounce fresh *or* frozen salmon steaks
4 cups water
⅓ cup lemon juice
1 small onion, sliced
¼ cup chopped celery
½ teaspoon salt
⅛ teaspoon freshly ground pepper
  Lemon wedges
  Tartar Sauce (see recipe, below) (optional)

Thaw salmon, if frozen. In large skillet combine water, lemon juice, onion, celery, salt, and pepper. Bring to boil; simmer 5 minutes. Add salmon; simmer, covered, 7 to 10 minutes or till fish flakes easily with a fork. Remove salmon from liquid with spatula. Chill or serve hot. Serve salmon with lemon wedges. If desired, top salmon with Tartar Sauce and garnish with fresh dillweed. Makes 4 servings. One serving (1 salmon steak) equals:

● ● ● ●   4 Lean Meat Exchanges

Tartar Sauce
pictured on page 64

½ cup whipped mayonnaise-type salad
    dressing substitute (no more than 20
    calories per tablespoon)
¼ cup finely shredded carrot
1 tablespoon finely chopped dill pickle
1 teaspoon finely chopped onion
1 teaspoon snipped parsley
1 teaspoon finely chopped pimiento
1 teaspoon lemon juice

Combine salad dressing, carrot, dill pickle, onion, parsley, pimiento, and lemon juice. Cover and chill thoroughly. Serve with fish. Makes ¾ cup sauce. One serving (2 tablespoons) equals:

◖   ½ Fat Exchange

Fish Creole

16 ounces fresh *or* frozen fish fillets
⅓ cup chopped onion
⅓ cup chopped green pepper
1 clove garlic, minced
1 16-ounce can tomatoes, cut up
2 tablespoons snipped parsley
1 tablespoon instant chicken bouillon granules
Dash bottled hot pepper sauce
1 tablespoon cornstarch
3 cups hot cooked rice

Thaw fish, if frozen. Cut into 1-inch cubes. Combine onion, green pepper, garlic, and 2 tablespoons *water*. Cook, covered, till tender. Add *undrained* tomatoes, parsley, bouillon, hot pepper sauce, and ½ cup *water*. Simmer, covered, 10 minutes. Blend cornstarch and 3 tablespoons cold *water*; stir into tomato mixture. Cook and stir till thickened. Stir in fish. Simmer, covered, 5 to 7 minutes. Serve over rice. Makes 6 servings. One serving (⅔ cup fish mixture and ½ cup rice) equals:

  2½ Lean Meat Exchanges

● 1 Bread Exchange

● 1 Vegetable Exchange

Oven Fried Fish a la Orange

1 pound fresh *or* frozen fish fillets
1 slightly beaten egg
½ of a 6-ounce can (6 tablespoons) frozen orange juice concentrate, thawed
2 tablespoons soy sauce
½ cup fine dry bread crumbs
2 tablespoons diet imitation margarine
½ teaspoon lemon juice

Thaw fish, if frozen. Combine next 3 ingredients. Combine crumbs and 1 teaspoon *salt*. Dip fish in egg mixture, then in crumb mixture. Place skin side down in 12x7½x2-inch baking dish. Melt margarine; stir in lemon juice. Drizzle over fish. Bake in 500° oven 10 to 12 minutes. Makes 4 servings. One serving (4 ounces) equals:

  4 Lean Meat Exchanges

● 1 Bread Exchange

○ 1 Fruit Exchange

● 1 Fat Exchange

Tuna Noodle Newburg

1 10¾-ounce can condensed cream of celery soup
⅔ cup evaporated skim milk
½ cup shredded low-calorie process cheese product (2 ounces)
⅓ cup whipped mayonnaise-type salad dressing substitute (no more than 20 calories per tablespoon)
¼ cup dry sherry
2 7-ounce cans water-pack tuna, drained
4 ounces medium noodles, cooked
1 cup thinly sliced celery
¼ cup chopped pimiento

Combine soup and evaporated milk. Bring to boil; stir often. Remove from heat; stir in cheese, salad dressing, and ¼ teaspoon *salt*. Stir till cheese melts. Blend in sherry. Add remaining ingredients; mix well. Turn into 1½-quart casserole. Bake, covered, in 350° oven 25 minutes. Makes 6 servings.

●●◖ 2½ Lean Meat Exchanges

● 1 Bread Exchange

● 1 Vegetable Exchange

◖ ½ Milk Exchange

Hearty Salmon Pie

1 tablespoon diet imitation margarine
2 cups soft bread crumbs (2½ slices bread)
⅔ cup skim milk
1 slightly beaten egg
2 tablespoons chopped onion
1 16-ounce can salmon, drained, boned, and finely flaked
3 hard-cooked eggs, chopped
2 cups plain mashed potatoes
3 tablespoons skim milk
1 egg

Melt margarine; stir in crumbs, ⅔ cup milk, 1 egg, onion, and ½ teaspoon *salt*. Stir in salmon and hard-cooked eggs. Turn into 9-inch pie plate. Combine potatoes and 3 tablespoons milk. Beat in remaining egg and 1 teaspoon *salt*. Spoon around edge of pie. Bake in 350° oven 30 to 35 minutes. Makes 6 servings. One serving (1/6 pie) equals:

  3 Lean Meat Exchanges

  1½ Bread Exchanges

Elegant Eggs Florentine

½ cup sliced green onion
2 tablespoons diet imitation margarine
6 tablespoons dry white wine
2 tablespoons vinegar
2 tablespoons diet imitation margarine
2 tablespoons cornstarch
2 cups skim milk
¼ teaspoon salt
¼ teaspoon dried tarragon, crushed
1 10-ounce package frozen chopped spinach, cooked and drained
1 4-ounce can sliced mushrooms, drained
3 small English muffins, split and toasted
6 tomato slices
6 eggs

In small saucepan cook onion in 2 tablespoons margarine till tender. Add dry white wine and vinegar. Simmer, reducing liquid by half. Meanwhile, in medium saucepan melt 2 tablespoons margarine. Blend in cornstarch. Add skim milk. Cook and stir till mixture is thickened and bubbly. Remove from heat; stir in salt and tarragon. Return to low heat; *gradually* stir in onion mixture. Add ¾ cup sauce mixture to cooked spinach; keep remaining sauce warm over low heat *(do not boil)*. Stir mushrooms into spinach mixture. Spoon ⅓ *cup* of the spinach mixture onto each toasted English muffin half. Top with 1 tomato slice. Broil 3 inches from heat about 5 minutes or till heated through; keep warm. Meanwhile, poach eggs in simmering water to desired doneness. Place poached eggs atop tomato slices. Top each egg with 3 tablespoons sauce. Makes 6 servings. One serving equals:

- ● 1 Lean Meat Exchange
- ● 1 Bread Exchange
- (½ Vegetable Exchange
- (½ Milk Exchange
- ●(1½ Fat Exchanges

Confetti Cheese Quiche
pictured on page 42

⅔ cup all-purpose flour
¼ teaspoon salt
3 tablespoons shortening
⅓ cup lowfat cottage cheese (no more than 2% butterfat), sieved
1 8½-ounce can mixed vegetables, drained
¼ cup finely chopped green onion
1 cup shredded low-calorie process cheese product (4 ounces)
3 slightly beaten eggs
1 cup evaporated skim milk
½ teaspoon salt
⅛ teaspoon pepper

In small bowl combine flour and ¼ teaspoon salt; cut in shortening till pieces are the size of small peas. Add cottage cheese. Toss mixture with fork till entire mixture is moistened. Form dough into a ball. Flatten on a very lightly floured surface by pressing with edge of hands 3 times across in both directions. Roll out to ⅛-inch thickness. Fit into a 9-inch pie plate or quiche pan; flute edges and set aside. In small bowl combine drained vegetables and onion. In cottage cheese pastry shell layer *half* the shredded cheese and the entire vegetable mixture. In large bowl combine slightly beaten eggs, evaporated skim milk, ½ teaspoon salt, and pepper. Pour egg mixture over vegetables in pastry shell. Sprinkle with remaining cheese. Bake in 325° oven 45 to 50 minutes or till knife inserted off-center comes out clean. Remove from oven and let stand 10 minutes before serving. (Texture may be soft.) Makes 8 servings. One serving (⅛ quiche) equals:

- ● 1 Lean Meat Exchange
- ● 1 Bread Exchange
- (½ Vegetable Exchange
- ● 1 Fat Exchange

Fruity Ham Sandwiches
pictured on page 50

½ cup whipped mayonnaise-type salad
   dressing substitute (no more than 20
   calories per tablespoon)
2 tablespoons chili sauce
1 tablespoon finely chopped dill pickle
2 teaspoons skim milk
4 slices whole wheat bread, toasted
   Lettuce
4 1-ounce slices Swiss cheese
4 1-ounce slices boiled ham
8 cantaloupe slices *or* 1 16-ounce can peach
   slices (juice pack), drained

Combine first 4 ingredients. Layer each slice of
toasted bread with lettuce, *1 tablespoon* dressing
mixture, cheese, ham, and ¼ cantaloupe or peach
slices. Drizzle with remaining dressing mixture.
Serves 4. One serving (1 sandwich) equals:

●● 2 Lean Meat Exchanges

●◖ 1½ Bread Exchanges

○ 1 Fruit Exchange

●● 2 Fat Exchanges

Vegetarian Sprout Sandwiches

1 cup thinly sliced cucumber
½ cup shredded carrot
2 tablespoons chopped green onion
⅓ cup low-calorie Italian salad dressing (no
   more than 8 calories per tablespoon)
4 ⅔-ounce slices low-calorie process cheese
   product
2 small English muffins, split and toasted
½ cup alfalfa sprouts
4 teaspoons shelled sunflower seed

Combine first 4 ingredients; set aside. Place 1
cheese slice atop each muffin half. Broil 5 inches
from heat for 2 minutes. Spoon ⅓ *cup* of vegetable
mixture atop each half; add *2 tablespoons* of the
sprouts and *1 teaspoon* of the sunflower seed.
Serves 4. One serving (1 sandwich) equals:

● 1 Lean Meat Exchange

● 1 Bread Exchange

● 1 Vegetable Exchange

Corned Beef Slaw-Wiches

½ cup whipped mayonnaise-type salad
   dressing substitute (no more than 20
   calories per tablespoon)
2 teaspoons prepared mustard
4 cups finely shredded cabbage
2 tablespoons sliced green onion
12 slices very thin whole wheat bread, toasted
1 12-ounce can corned beef, chilled

Blend salad dressing and mustard. Combine cabbage and onion; toss with salad dressing mixture.
Spoon ½ *cup* of cabbage mixture onto 6 of the
toasted bread slices. Cut corned beef into 12
slices; arrange 2 slices atop each sandwich. Top
with remaining toasted bread. Serves 6. One serving (1 sandwich) equals:

●● 2 Lean Meat Exchanges

● 1 Bread Exchange

◖ ½ Vegetable Exchange

●● 2 Fat Exchanges

Turkey-Asparagus Stacks
pictured on the cover

¼ cup low-calorie French salad dressing (no
   more than 25 calories per tablespoon)
2 tablespoons finely chopped onion
1 10-ounce package frozen asparagus spears,
   cooked and drained
2 bagels, halved and toasted
8 1-ounce slices cooked turkey
4 ⅔-ounce slices low-calorie process cheese
   product, halved diagonally

Combine salad dressing, onion, and ⅛ teaspoon
pepper; pour over asparagus. Refrigerate several
hours. Remove asparagus with slotted spoon.
Spread some dressing mixture on bagels. Top with
turkey; spread dressing mixture between turkey
slices. Top with asparagus. Broil 4 inches from heat
4 minutes. Place cheese atop asparagus. Broil 1
minute more. Makes 4 servings. One serving (1
sandwich) equals:

●●◖ 2½ Lean Meat Exchanges

● 1 Bread Exchange

● 1 Vegetable Exchange

◖ ½ Fat Exchange

salads and vegetables

Cucumber Cheese Mold

- 1 envelope unflavored gelatin
- 1½ cups chicken broth
- 1 tablespoon lemon juice
- 1½ teaspoons prepared horseradish
- ¼ cup thinly sliced cucumber
- 1½ cups dry cottage cheese (12 ounces)
- ⅓ cup seeded, shredded cucumber
- ⅓ cup shredded carrot
- 2 tablespoons chopped green onion

Soften gelatin in broth. Add lemon juice and horseradish; stir over low heat till dissolved. Cool. Arrange cucumber slices in 4-cup mold. Pour ½ cup gelatin mixture into mold. Chill till almost firm. Combine remaining gelatin mixture with remaining ingredients. Turn into mold. Chill till firm. Makes 6 servings. One serving (about ⅔ cup) equals:

- ● 1 Lean Meat Exchange
- ◖ ½ Vegetable Exchange

Sparkling Citrus Mold

- 1 8-ounce can grapefruit sections (juice pack)
  Orange juice
- 1 envelope unflavored gelatin
- 1 cup low-calorie orange carbonated beverage, chilled
- 1 tablespoon lemon juice
- ½ cup orange sections

Drain grapefruit, reserving juice. Add enough orange juice to reserved juice to measure 1 cup; soften gelatin in juice mixture. Stir over low heat till dissolved. Add orange beverage and lemon juice. Chill till partially set (consistency of unbeaten egg whites). Cut up orange and grapefruit sections; fold into gelatin. Turn into 3-cup mold. Chill till firm. Makes 4 servings. One serving (¾ cup) equals:

- ● 1 Fruit Exchange

Molded Gazpacho Salad

- 1 4-serving envelope low-calorie lemon-flavored gelatin
- ¾ cup vegetable juice cocktail
- 2 tablespoons low-calorie Italian salad dressing (no more than 8 calories per tablespoon)
- 4 teaspoons vinegar
- ½ cup sliced cauliflowerets
- ½ cup chopped, seeded tomato
- ½ cup chopped celery
- ¼ cup chopped green pepper

Dissolve gelatin in ¾ cup boiling *water*. Stir in vegetable juice, salad dressing, and vinegar. Chill till partially set (consistency of unbeaten egg whites). Fold in remaining ingredients. Turn into 3-cup mold. Chill several hours or till firm. Makes 4 servings. One serving (about ⅔ cup) equals:

- ● 1 Vegetable Exchange

Shimmering Iceberg Rings

- 1 4-serving envelope low-calorie lime-flavored gelatin
- 1 tablespoon vinegar
- 1½ cups chopped iceberg lettuce
- ¼ cup finely chopped radish

Dissolve gelatin and ¼ teaspoon *salt* in 1 cup boiling *water*. Stir in ⅔ cup cold *water* and vinegar. Chill till partially set (consistency of unbeaten egg whites). Fold in lettuce and radish. Turn into 4 individual molds. Chill several hours or till firm. Makes 4 servings. One serving (½ cup) equals:

- ● 1 Free Exchange

Cucumber Cheese Mold, top, and Carrot-Potato Boats, bottom (see recipe, page 75).

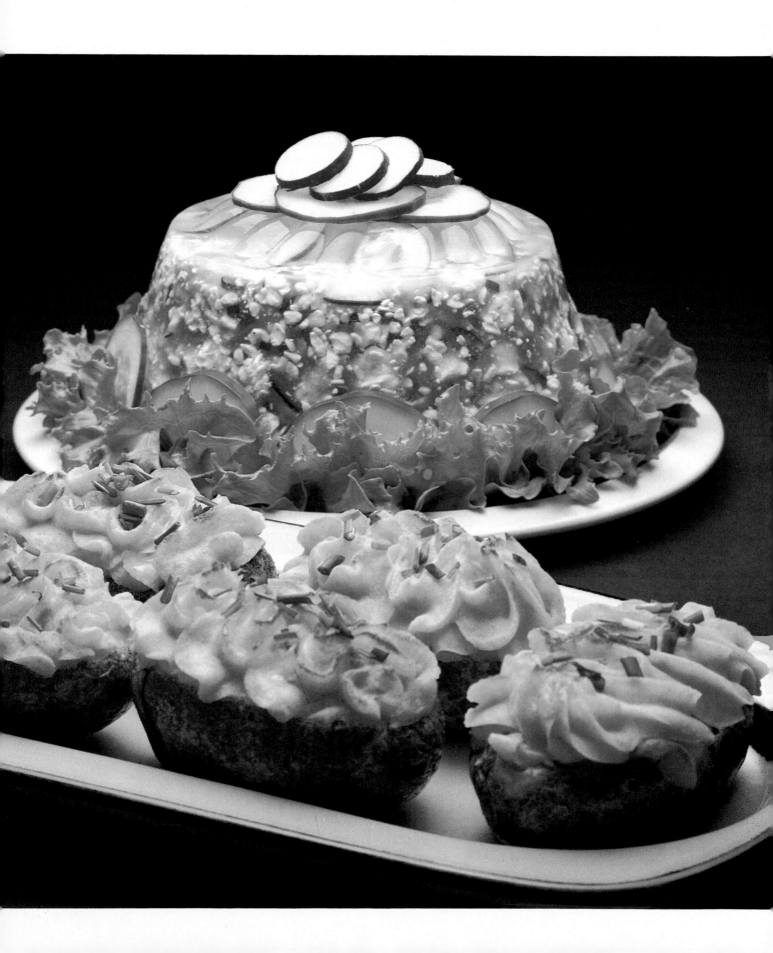

Tangy Vegetable Vinaigrette

    1 tablespoon cornstarch
    1 teaspoon dry mustard
    1 cup cold water
    ¼ cup vinegar
    ¼ cup catsup
    1 teaspoon worcestershire sauce
    ½ teaspoon salt
    ½ teaspoon prepared horseradish
    ¼ teaspoon paprika
    ⅛ teaspoon garlic powder
    1 cup thinly sliced cauliflowerets
    1 cup thinly sliced carrot
    1 cup thinly sliced cucumber
    1 cup thinly sliced celery
    ¼ cup thinly sliced green onion
      Lettuce

Combine cornstarch and dry mustard; gradually stir in cold water. Cook and stir till thickened and bubbly. Remove from heat. Cover surface with waxed paper. Cool 10 to 15 minutes. Stir in vinegar, catsup, worcestershire sauce, salt, horseradish, paprika, and garlic powder. In large bowl combine cauliflowerets, carrot, cucumber, celery, and green onion. Add dressing; stir gently. Cover; refrigerate several hours or overnight, stirring occasionally. To serve, drain vegetables; mound in lettuce-lined bowl. Makes 8 servings. One serving (½ cup) equals:

● 1 Vegetable Exchange

Calorie Counter's Coleslaw

    2 cups shredded cabbage
    ¾ cup shredded carrot
    ¼ cup thinly sliced bermuda onion
    ½ cup lowfat plain yogurt (no more than 2% butterfat)
    2 teaspoons cooking oil
    1 teaspoon prepared horseradish

Combine cabbage, carrot, and onion. Stir together yogurt, oil, horseradish, ⅛ teaspoon *salt,* and dash *pepper.* Toss yogurt mixture with cabbage mixture to coat. Chill several hours. Makes 4 servings. One serving (¾ cup) equals:

● 1 Vegetable Exchange
● 1 Fat Exchange

Layered Vegetable Salad
pictured on page 50

    1 small head lettuce, torn into pieces
    2 small bermuda onions, thinly sliced and separated into rings
    2 cups thinly sliced zucchini
    2 cups cherry tomatoes, halved
    ½ of an 8-ounce package neufchatel cheese, softened
    1 teaspoon worcestershire sauce
    ½ teaspoon dry mustard
    1 cup lowfat plain yogurt (no more than 2% butterfat)

In salad bowl layer lettuce, onions, zucchini, and cherry tomatoes. To prepare dressing, combine cheese, worcestershire sauce, and mustard. Stir in yogurt. Spoon dressing over vegetables in bowl. If desired, sprinkle with paprika. Cover; refrigerate 4 to 6 hours or overnight. Toss just before serving. Makes 8 servings. One serving (1¼ cups) equals:

◖ ½ Lean Meat Exchange
● 1 Vegetable Exchange
◖ ½ Fat Exchange

Spinach Salad Toss

    2 tablespoons cooking oil
    1 teaspoon sesame seed, toasted
    ½ teaspoon finely shredded lime peel
    4 teaspoons lime juice
    ¼ teaspoon dry mustard
    ⅛ teaspoon salt
    3 cups torn fresh spinach
    1 cup sliced fresh mushrooms
    ½ cup sliced radishes
    2 hard-cooked eggs, sliced

For dressing, in small screw-top jar combine oil, sesame seed, lime peel, lime juice, mustard, and salt. Cover and shake well; chill. To serve, combine spinach, mushrooms, radishes, and egg slices. Shake dressing and toss with spinach mixture. Makes 4 servings. One serving (1½ cups) equals:

◖ ½ Lean Meat Exchange
◖ ½ Vegetable Exchange
●● 2 Fat Exchanges

Tijuana Taco Salad

1 pound ground beef (15% fat)
¼ cup chopped onion
1 7½-ounce can tomatoes, cut up
2 teaspoons chili powder
¼ teaspoon garlic powder
¼ teaspoon salt
⅛ teaspoon ground cumin
⅛ teaspoon pepper
1 large head lettuce
3 medium tomatoes, cut into wedges
¾ cup shredded low-calorie process cheese
    product (3 ounces)

Cook beef and onion till beef is browned; drain. Stir in *undrained* tomatoes, chili powder, garlic powder, salt, cumin, and pepper. Bring to boil; simmer till most liquid evaporates, stirring occasionally. Line 6 individual salad bowls with large lettuce leaves; tear remainder into bite-size pieces and divide among salad bowls. Spoon beef mixture onto lettuce. Arrange tomatoes atop; sprinkle with cheese. Makes 6 servings. One serving (1 salad) equals:

● ● ◖   2½ Lean Meat Exchanges
   ●   1 Vegetable Exchange
   ●   1 Fat Exchange

Seafaring Salmon Salad

1 7¾-ounce can salmon, drained, boned, and
    flaked
1 tablespoon lemon juice
2 hard-cooked eggs, coarsely chopped
¼ cup thinly sliced dill pickle
¼ cup whipped mayonnaise-type salad
    dressing substitute (no more than 20
    calories per tablespoon)
2 tablespoons sliced green onion
¼ teaspoon salt
    Dash pepper

Sprinkle salmon with lemon juice; stir in hard-cooked eggs, pickle, salad dressing, green onion, salt, and pepper. Mix gently and chill. If desired, serve on lettuce-lined plates. Makes 4 servings. One serving (⅓ cup) equals:

● ●   2 Lean Meat Exchanges
 ●   1 Vegetable Exchange
 ◖   ½ Fat Exchange

Chef's Salad Bowl

1½ cups thinly sliced cauliflowerets
1 cup sliced radishes
½ cup sliced green onion
½ cup low-calorie French salad dressing (no
    more than 25 calories per tablespoon)
4 cups torn mixed salad greens
4 ounces low-calorie process cheese product,
    cut into julienne strips
4 ounces fully cooked center-cut ham, cut
    into julienne strips
8 cherry tomatoes, halved
4 hard-cooked eggs, quartered

Combine cauliflowerets, radishes, and green onion. Add French salad dressing; toss. Refrigerate 4 hours, tossing occasionally. Place salad greens in 4 individual salad bowls. Arrange cheese, ham, cherry tomatoes, and eggs atop greens. To serve, drain vegetable mixture; reserve dressing. Spoon some of the vegetable mixture atop each salad. Drizzle with reserved dressing. Makes 4 servings. One serving (1 salad) equals:

● ● ●   3 Lean Meat Exchanges
 ● ●   2 Vegetable Exchanges
  ●   1 Fat Exchange

Trimming Tuna Toss

¾ cup wine vinegar
1½ teaspoons dried basil, crushed
¼ teaspoon salt
    Dash pepper
2 7-ounce cans water-pack tuna, drained
8 cups torn lettuce
1½ cups cherry tomatoes, halved
1 medium cucumber, sliced
½ medium onion, thinly sliced and separated
    into rings
½ cup sliced celery

Combine vinegar, basil, salt, and pepper; chill. In large salad bowl break up tuna; add lettuce, cherry tomatoes, cucumber, onion, and celery. Add vinegar mixture and toss lightly. Makes 7 servings. One serving (1¾ cups) equals:

● ◖   1½ Lean Meat Exchanges
 ◖   ½ Vegetable Exchange

Chicken-Stuffed Oranges

4 large oranges
1 cup thinly sliced celery
¼ cup orange yogurt
1 tablespoon thinly sliced green onion
½ teaspoon celery salt
1⅓ cups diced cooked chicken (8 ounces)

Cut tops off oranges; remove fruit and chop. Chill orange shells. Combine chopped orange, celery, yogurt, onion, and celery salt. To serve, stir chicken into orange mixture; spoon mixture into shells. Serves 4. One serving (1 stuffed orange) equals:

⬤⬤ 2 Lean Meat Exchanges
◯ 1 Fruit Exchange
⬤ 1 Vegetable Exchange

Zippy Waldorf Salad

3 medium apples, cored and chopped
½ cup chopped celery
½ cup apple yogurt
⅓ cup seeded, halved red grapes
¼ cup chopped walnuts

Combine all ingredients. Cover; chill 2 to 3 hours. If desired, turn into a romaine-lined bowl. Makes 8 servings. One serving (½ cup) equals:

◯ 1 Fruit Exchange
◖ ½ Fat Exchange

Tangy Tomato Dressing
pictured on page 42

2 teaspoons cornstarch
1 cup vegetable juice cocktail
¼ cup chili sauce
1 tablespoon cooking oil
1 tablespoon lime *or* lemon juice
2 teaspoons prepared horseradish

Combine cornstarch and ¼ teaspoon *salt*. Add vegetable juice. Cook and stir till thickened; cook 1 minute more. Stir in remaining ingredients. Cover; chill. Makes 1⅓ cups. One serving (2 tablespoons) equals:

◖ ½ Vegetable Exchange

Blue Cheese Dressing

1 cup lowfat cottage cheese (no more than 2% butterfat)
⅓ cup crumbled blue cheese
4 teaspoons lemon juice
½ cup skim milk

In blender container combine cottage cheese, *half* the blue cheese, and lemon juice. Cover; blend till creamy. Blend in skim milk a tablespoon at a time. Stir in remaining blue cheese. Cover; chill. Serve with vegetable or fruit salads. Makes 1⅔ cups. One serving (2 tablespoons) equals:

◖ ½ Lean Meat Exchange
◣ ¼ Fat Exchange

Potluck Potato Salad

5 medium potatoes
¼ cup low-calorie French salad dressing (no more than 25 calories per tablespoon)
1 cup chopped celery
⅓ cup chopped onion
4 hard-cooked eggs, sliced
1 teaspoon salt
1 teaspoon celery seed
½ cup whipped mayonnaise-type salad dressing substitute (no more than 20 calories per tablespoon)
2 teaspoons prepared mustard
½ to 1 teaspoon prepared horseradish

Cook unpeeled potatoes till tender in boiling water; peel and cube. Combine warm potatoes and French salad dressing; toss gently to coat. Chill 2 hours. Add celery, onion, eggs, salt, and celery seed. Combine salad dressing substitute, mustard, and horseradish; toss gently with potato mixture. Chill 4 hours. Makes 8 servings. One serving (¾ cup) equals:

◖ ½ Lean Meat Exchange
⬤ 1 Bread Exchange
◖ ½ Vegetable Exchange
◖ ½ Fat Exchange

Carrot-Potato Boats
pictured on page 71

- **4 small baking potatoes**
- **½ of an 8-ounce package neufchatel cheese, cut into chunks and softened**
- **3 to 4 tablespoons skim milk**
- **¼ teaspoon salt**
  Dash pepper
- **1 cup cooked chopped carrot, pureed**
- **2 tablespoons chopped green onion**

Bake potatoes in 375° oven 45 minutes or till done. Cool slightly; cut potatoes in half lengthwise. Scoop out potatoes into small mixer bowl, reserving shells. Add neufchatel cheese, milk, salt, and pepper. Beat till fluffy, adding more milk if necessary. Fold in carrot and green onion. Pipe or spoon potato mixture into potato shells. Bake on a baking sheet in 375° oven 12 to 15 minutes or till heated through. If desired, sprinkle with chives. Makes 8 servings. One serving (1 potato boat) equals:

- ◖ ½ Lean Meat Exchange
- ● 1 Bread Exchange

Creamy Spinach Custard

- **8 ounces fresh spinach (6 cups)**
- **2 eggs**
- **1 cup skim milk**
- **¼ teaspoon ground nutmeg**
- **½ cup shredded monterey jack cheese (2 ounces)**

Cook spinach in small amount of lightly salted boiling water 3 to 5 minutes or till tender; drain well. Chop coarsely; pat between paper toweling to remove excess liquid. Beat eggs, skim milk, nutmeg, and ½ teaspoon *salt* till blended. Stir in cheese and spinach. Turn into four 6-ounce custard cups. Set cups in shallow baking pan on oven rack. Pour hot water into pan to depth of 1 inch. Bake in 350° oven 35 to 40 minutes. Remove from water; let stand 5 minutes before serving. Makes 4 servings. One serving (1 custard) equals:

- ● 1 Lean Meat Exchange
- ● 1 Vegetable Exchange
- ◣ ¼ Milk Exchange
- ◖ ½ Fat Exchange

Vegetable Skillet

- **4 cups thinly sliced zucchini**
- **1 cup coarsely shredded carrot**
- **1 cup chopped onion**
- **¾ cup bias-sliced celery**
- **½ medium green pepper, cut into thin strips**
- **½ teaspoon garlic salt**
- **¼ teaspoon dried basil, crushed**
  Dash pepper
- **2 tablespoons cooking oil**
- **¼ cup chili sauce**
- **2 teaspoons prepared mustard**
- **2 medium tomatoes, cut into wedges**

In large skillet cook zucchini, carrot, onion, celery, green pepper, garlic salt, basil, and pepper, covered, in hot oil over medium-high heat 4 minutes, stirring occasionally. Combine chili sauce and mustard; stir into vegetable mixture. Add tomato wedges; cook 2 to 3 minutes or till heated through. Season to taste with salt. Serve in skillet or transfer to serving dish. Makes 8 servings. One serving (¾ cup) equals:

- 1½ Vegetable Exchanges
- ● 1 Fat Exchange

Bean-Stuffed Tomatoes

- **1 9-ounce package frozen Italian *or* cut green beans, cooked and drained**
- **1 2½-ounce jar sliced mushrooms, drained**
- **⅓ cup low-calorie Italian salad dressing (no more than 8 calories per tablespoon)**
- **¼ cup sliced green onion**
- **¼ teaspoon salt**
  Dash pepper
- **6 medium tomatoes**

Combine beans, mushrooms, salad dressing, green onion, salt, and pepper; toss. Refrigerate 2 hours, tossing occasionally. Cut tops off tomatoes; scoop out pulp, leaving ¼-inch shells. (Reserve pulp for another use.) Invert shells on paper toweling; chill. To serve, season shells to taste with *salt;* fill with bean mixture. Makes 6 servings. One serving (1 stuffed tomato) equals:

- 1½ Vegetable Exchanges

desserts

Strawberry Ribbon Pie

¾ cup finely crushed graham crackers
   (11 crackers)
2 tablespoons diet imitation margarine,
   melted
1 ⅝-ounce package (2 envelopes) low-calorie
   strawberry-flavored gelatin
1 tablespoon lemon juice
2 cups fresh *or* frozen whole unsweetened
   strawberries, thawed
2 eggs whites
¼ teaspoon cream of tartar
1 1¼-ounce envelope low-calorie dessert
   topping mix
1 teaspoon skim milk

Combine graham cracker crumbs and margarine. Press mixture firmly into 9-inch pie plate. Chill. Dissolve gelatin in 2 cups boiling *water;* add lemon juice. Measure ½ *cup* of gelatin mixture; stir in ½ cup cold *water.* Chill till partially set (consistency of unbeaten egg whites). Turn into chilled graham cracker crust; chill till almost firm.

To remaining gelatin mixture add ½ cup cold *water* and chill till partially set. Reserve a few strawberries for garnish. Sieve remaining strawberries; fold into partially set gelatin. In small mixer bowl beat egg whites with cream of tartar till stiff peaks form. Prepare dessert topping mix according to package directions. Gently fold egg whites into partially set gelatin mixture. Fold in ¾ *cup* of whipped topping. (Refrigerate remaining topping.) If necessary, chill strawberry mixture till it mounds. Pile strawberry mixture atop first layer in crust. Chill till firm. Stir skim milk into remaining topping till smooth and fluffy. Pipe or spoon whipped topping around edge of pie. Garnish with reserved strawberries. Makes 8 servings. One serving (⅛ pie) equals:

◖ ½ Bread Exchange

◖ ½ Fruit Exchange

● 1 Fat Exchange

Pineapple Dream Pie
pictured on the cover

¾ cup flaked coconut
1 tablespoon diet imitation margarine, melted
1 4-serving-size envelope *regular* low-calorie
   vanilla pudding mix
1 20-ounce can crushed pineapple (juice
   pack)
1 envelope unflavored gelatin
2 tablespoons lemon juice
½ cup whipped low-calorie dessert topping

In small bowl combine flaked coconut and margarine; press on bottom and sides of 9-inch pie plate. Bake coconut pie shell in 325° oven about 15 minutes or till golden; cool.

Prepare pudding mix according to package directions. Cover surface of pudding with waxed paper; cool to room temperature. Meanwhile, drain pineapple; reserve juice in 1-cup measure. Add water to juice to equal ¾ cup. Soften gelatin in pineapple juice mixture. Stir over low heat till gelatin is dissolved; stir in lemon juice. Chill gelatin mixture till partially set (consistency of unbeaten egg whites). Whip partially set gelatin till fluffy; fold in cooled pudding and 1¼ *cups* of the crushed pineapple. (Reserve remainder for another use.) Pour pineapple mixture into cooled pie shell. Garnish pie with dollops of whipped low-calorie dessert topping. Makes 8 servings. One serving (⅛ pie) equals:

◐ 1 Fruit Exchange

◖ ½ Milk Exchange

● 1 Fat Exchange

*Ribbon Mocha Parfaits, top left (see recipe, page 80);
Ruby Fruit Compote, top right (see recipe, page 80); and
Strawberry Ribbon Pie, bottom.*

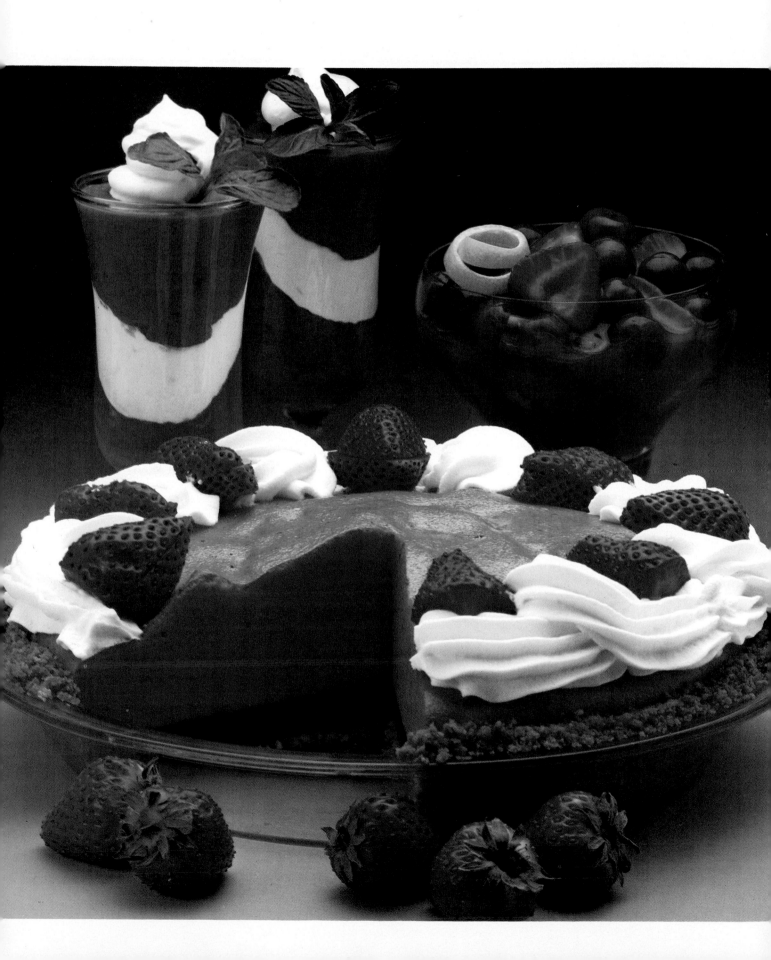

Mint Chocolate Cream Puffs

       2 tablespoons butter *or* margarine
       ½ cup boiling water
       ½ cup all-purpose flour
       ⅛ teaspoon salt
       2 eggs
       1 4-serving-size envelope *regular* low-calorie
          chocolate pudding mix
       ¼ teaspoon peppermint extract
       1 1¼-ounce envelope low-calorie dessert
          topping mix

In small saucepan melt butter or margarine in boiling water. Add flour and salt all at once; stir vigorously. Cook and stir till mixture forms a ball that does not separate. Remove from heat; cool 5 minutes. Add eggs one at a time, beating till dough is very smooth and shiny after each addition. Drop dough 3 inches apart on lightly greased baking sheet, making 8 mounds. Bake in 450° oven 15 minutes. Reduce heat to 325°. Bake 10 minutes more. Remove cream puffs from oven; cut off tops. Remove soft centers. Turn oven off; return hollow cream puff tops and bottoms to oven for 20 minutes to dry. Cool cream puffs on a wire rack.

Meanwhile, in medium saucepan prepare the chocolate pudding mix according to package directions. Stir in peppermint extract. Cover surface of the chocolate pudding with waxed paper; cool the chocolate pudding to room temperature. In small mixer bowl prepare the dessert topping mix according to package directions. Stir the chocolate pudding; fold the whipped topping into the chocolate pudding. Cover; chill.

Spoon about ½ *cup* of the chilled chocolate pudding mixture into each of the cream puff bottoms. Top with the cream puff tops. One serving (1 filled cream puff) equals:

   ◖ ½ Bread Exchange

   ◖ ½ Milk Exchange

   ●● 2 Fat Exchanges

Pumpkin-Spice Cake

       2¼ cups sifted cake flour
       1 tablespoon baking powder
       1½ teaspoons ground cinnamon
       ¾ teaspoon ground cloves
       ¾ teaspoon ground nutmeg
       7 eggs, separated
       ½ of a 16-ounce can (1 cup) pumpkin
       ½ cup cooking oil
          Non-caloric liquid sweetener equal to ½ cup
          sugar
       ½ teaspoon finely shredded orange peel
       ½ teaspoon cream of tartar
       1 1¼-ounce envelope low-calorie dessert
          topping mix, whipped

Sift together flour, baking powder, spices, and ¼ teaspoon *salt*. Combine egg yolks and next four ingredients; beat smooth. Wash beaters. Beat egg whites and cream of tartar to stiff peaks. Fold pumpkin mixture into whites. Sprinkle ¼ dry ingredients atop. Fold in dry ingredients, adding ¼ at a time. Turn into ungreased 9-inch tube pan. Bake in 325° oven 45 minutes. Invert in pan; cool. Remove; serve with topping. Serves 16. One serving (1/16 cake and 2 tablespoons topping) equals:

   ◖ ½ Lean Meat Exchange

   ● 1 Bread Exchange

   ●● 2 Fat Exchanges

Peach Fondue

       1 16-ounce can peach halves (juice pack)
       1 teaspoon cornstarch
       ¼ teaspoon ground cinnamon
       ⅛ teaspoon ground allspice
       ½ teaspoon vanilla
       1 cup cubed cantaloupe
       1 small apple, cored and cut into wedges
       ¾ cup fresh strawberries, hulled
       ½ small banana, cut into chunks

In blender container combine *undrained* peaches, cornstarch, cinnamon, and allspice. Cover; blend till nearly smooth. Pour into saucepan; cook and stir till thickened. Stir in vanilla. Transfer to fondue pot; keep warm over fondue burner. Serve with fruit as dippers. Makes 5 servings. One serving (¼ cup peach sauce and ⅕ fruit) equals:

   ●● 2 Fruit Exchanges

Orange Chiffon Soufflé

⅓ cup nonfat dry milk powder
2 tablespoons cornstarch
⅛ teaspoon salt
¾ cup water
1 teaspoon finely shredded orange peel
½ cup orange juice
Non-caloric liquid sweetener equal to
2 tablespoons sugar
5 egg yolks
5 egg whites
4 teaspoons cornstarch
Dash salt
Non-caloric liquid sweetener equal to
1 tablespoon sugar
1 medium orange
8 drops almond extract
Red and yellow food coloring (optional)

In saucepan combine nonfat dry milk, 2 tablespoons cornstarch, and ⅛ teaspoon salt. Gradually stir in water. Cook and stir till mixture is thickened and bubbly. Remove from heat; stir in orange peel, orange juice, and non-caloric sweetener equal to 2 tablespoons sugar. Beat egg yolks till thick and lemon-colored. Slowly add thickened orange mixture to egg yolks, stirring constantly. Wash beaters. Beat egg whites till stiff peaks form. Carefully fold egg yolk mixture into beaten egg whites. Gently pour mixture into ungreased 2-quart soufflé dish with a foil collar. Bake in 325° oven 65 to 70 minutes or till knife inserted off-center comes out clean. Meanwhile, for sauce, in small saucepan combine 4 teaspoons cornstarch, dash salt, and the remaining sweetener. Peel and section orange over bowl to catch juice; cut up sections. Add enough *water* to reserved juice to equal 1 cup. Blend orange juice mixture into cornstarch mixture. Cook and stir till mixture is thickened and bubbly. Remove from heat; stir in orange sections and almond extract. If desired, tint orange sauce with food coloring. To serve, spoon sauce over individual servings of warm soufflé. Makes 8 servings. One serving (⅛ soufflé and about 2 tablespoons sauce) equals:

● 1 Lean Meat Exchange
◗ 1 Fruit Exchange

Cranberry-Cherry Crepes

1½ cups frozen pitted tart red cherries
1 egg
⅔ cup skim milk
½ cup all-purpose flour
2 teaspoons butter *or* margarine, melted
½ cup dairy sour cream
⅛ teaspoon ground cinnamon
2 teaspoons cornstarch
Non-caloric liquid sweetener equal to
2 tablespoons sugar
¾ teaspoon finely shredded orange peel
1 cup low-calorie cranberry juice cocktail

Thaw frozen cherries. Combine egg, skim milk, flour, and butter or margarine; beat till smooth. Lightly grease 6-inch crepe pan; heat. Add 2 tablespoons batter; lift pan and tilt till batter covers bottom. Brown crepe on one side. Turn onto waxed paper. Repeat with remaining batter. Combine sour cream and cinnamon; spread unbrowned side of each crepe with *1 tablespoon* of mixture. Roll up; place in 13x9x2-inch baking dish. Combine cornstarch, sweetener, and peel. Stir in cranberry juice. Add cherries. Cook and stir till thickened; pour over crepes. Bake in 375° oven 15 minutes. Makes 8 servings. One serving (1 crepe and 3 tablespoons sauce) equals:

◖ ½ Bread Exchange
◗ 1 Fruit Exchange
● 1 Fat Exchange

Fresh Fruit Medley

3 ounces neufchatel cheese, softened
⅔ cup strawberry yogurt
2¼ cups fresh *or* frozen whole unsweetened
strawberries, thawed
2 small oranges, sectioned
2 small bananas, bias-sliced

In small mixer bowl beat cheese till fluffy. Add *half* the yogurt; beat till smooth. Stir in remaining yogurt. Cover; chill. Halve strawberries; combine with oranges and bananas. Chill. To serve, spoon ½ *cup* of fruit into each of 8 compotes; spoon yogurt mixture atop. Makes 8 servings. One serving (½ cup fruit and 2 tablespoons yogurt mixture) equals:

◖ ½ Lean Meat Exchange
◗◖ 1½ Fruit Exchanges

Ribbon Mocha Parfait
pictured on page 77

    1 4-serving-size envelope *regular* low-calorie
       chocolate pudding mix
    2 teaspoons instant coffee crystals
 1¾ cups skim milk
    2 stiff-beaten egg whites
    1 1¼-ounce envelope low-calorie dessert
       topping mix

Combine pudding mix and coffee crystals; slowly stir in skim milk. Cook and stir till thickened and bubbly. Remove from heat. Cover surface of pudding with waxed paper and cool to room temperature. Fold in egg whites. Prepare topping mix according to package directions. Fold ½ cup of the topping into pudding. Alternately spoon pudding and remaining topping into 6 parfait glasses. Chill. If desired, top with mint leaves. Makes 6 servings. One serving (1 parfait) equals:

◖ ½ Milk Exchange

● 1 Fat Exchange

Ruby Fruit Compote
pictured on page 77

    1 16-ounce package frozen pitted tart red
       cherries
    1 tablespoon cornstarch
       Non-caloric liquid sweetener equal to ½ cup
       sugar
       Dash salt
 1½ cups cold water
    1 tablespoon lemon juice
    4 drops red food coloring (optional)
    2 cups fresh *or* frozen whole unsweetened
       strawberries, thawed

Thaw frozen cherries. Combine cornstarch, sweetener, and salt. Blend water into cornstarch mixture. Cook and stir till thickened and bubbly. Add lemon juice and food coloring, if desired. Halve large strawberries. Stir strawberries and cherries into cornstarch mixture. Chill. To serve, spoon ½ cup of the fruit into each of 9 compotes. If desired, top with lemon peel twist. Makes 9 servings. One serving (½ cup fruit) equals:

◦ 1 Fruit Exchange

Tapioca Pudding Parfait
pictured on the cover

    2 cups skim milk
    2 tablespoons quick-cooking tapioca
       Non-caloric liquid sweetener equal to ¼ cup
       sugar
  ¼ teaspoon salt
    2 slightly beaten egg yolks
  ½ teaspoon vanilla
    2 egg whites
    6 cups fresh *or* frozen whole unsweetened
       strawberries, thawed

Combine skim milk, tapioca, sweetener, and salt. Let stand 5 minutes. Add egg yolks. Cook and stir till bubbly. Remove from heat (mixture will be thin); stir in vanilla. In small mixer bowl beat egg whites till soft peaks form. Gradually fold in hot mixture. Halve strawberries; reserve a few strawberries for garnish. Alternate layers of pudding with halved strawberries in 8 parfait glasses, ending with tapioca. Garnish with reserved strawberries. Chill. Makes 8 servings. One serving (1 parfait) equals:

◦ 1 Fruit Exchange

◖ ½ Milk Exchange

Banana Freeze
pictured on page 38

    1 4-serving-size envelope *regular* low-calorie
       vanilla pudding mix
  ¼ teaspoon almond extract
    2 small fully ripe bananas, mashed
    2 stiff-beaten egg whites
    5 maraschino cherries, halved

Prepare pudding mix according to package directions. Stir in extract. Cover surface of pudding with waxed paper; cool to room temperature. Fold in bananas and egg whites. Spoon into 10 paper bake cups in muffin pans. Freeze firm. Let stand at room temperature 30 minutes before serving. To serve, trim with cherries. Makes 10 servings. One serving (⅓ cup) equals:

◖ ½ Bread Exchange

◦ ½ Fruit Exchange

Molded Crème de Cinnamon

3 cups skim milk
  Non-caloric liquid sweetener equal to ¾ cup
    sugar
9 inches stick cinnamon, broken
2 envelopes unflavored gelatin
¼ cup cold water
1 cup dairy sour cream
1 teaspoon vanilla
  Peach-Berry Sauce (see recipe, below)
    (optional)

Combine skim milk, sweetener, and cinnamon. Cook over low heat 10 to 15 minutes, stirring occasionally. Remove cinnamon. Soften gelatin in cold water. Add to hot milk mixture; stir to dissolve. Chill till partially set (consistency of unbeaten egg whites). Combine sour cream and vanilla. Fold into gelatin mixture. Pour into 4-cup mold or 8 individual molds. Chill till firm. If desired, serve with Peach-Berry Sauce. Makes 8 servings. One serving (½ cup) equals:

◖ ½ Milk Exchange

● 1 Fat Exchange

Peach-Berry Sauce
pictured on page 46

1 16-ounce can peach slices (juice pack)
2 tablespoons water
2 teaspoons cornstarch
1 tablespoon peach brandy
¾ cup fresh or frozen whole unsweetened
    strawberries, thawed and halved
¼ teaspoon ground cinnamon
⅛ teaspoon ground allspice
  Molded Crème de Cinnamon (see recipe,
    above), waffles, or pancakes (optional)

Drain peaches; reserve juice. Blend water into cornstarch. Blend in reserved juice and peach brandy. Cook and stir till thickened and bubbly; stir in the peaches, strawberries, cinnamon, and allspice. Heat through. If desired, serve atop Molded Crème de Cinnamon, waffles, or pancakes. Makes 8 servings. One serving (about ⅓ cup) equals:

◐ 1 Fruit Exchange

Plum Whip

1 envelope unflavored gelatin
¼ cup cold water
1 16-ounce can dietetic-pack red plums
    (artificially sweetened)
1 tablespoon lemon juice
6 to 8 drops red food coloring (optional)
2 egg whites
  Dash salt
1 1¼-ounce envelope low-calorie dessert
    topping mix

Soften gelatin in cold water. Sieve *undrained* plums into saucepan; bring to boil. Stir in softened gelatin and lemon juice. Add food coloring, if desired. Stir till dissolved. Chill till partially set (consistency of unbeaten egg whites). In large mixer bowl beat egg whites with salt till soft peaks form; gradually add plum mixture and beat till fluffy. Prepare topping mix according to package directions; fold *half* into plum mixture. Chill till partially set. Mound into individual serving dishes; chill. Use remaining topping as garnish. Makes 6 servings. One serving (about ½ cup) equals:

◐ 1 Fruit Exchange

● 1 Fat Exchange

Layered Peach Dessert
pictured on page 50

1 4-serving envelope low-calorie lemon- *or*
    raspberry-flavored gelatin
¾ cup boiling water
¾ cup cold water
1 16-ounce can peach slices (juice pack),
    drained and cut up
¼ cup chilled evaporated skim milk
  Few drops almond extract

Dissolve gelatin in boiling water. Stir in cold water. Add *1 cup* of the gelatin mixture to peaches; chill till partially set. Chill remaining gelatin till partially set (consistency of unbeaten egg whites). Add evaporated skim milk and almond extract to partially set gelatin *without* peaches. Beat till fluffy. In 6 parfait glasses layer the 2 gelatin mixtures, ending with whipped gelatin. Chill thoroughly before serving. Makes 6 servings. One serving (1 parfait) equals:

◐ 1 Fruit Exchange

family-style reducing

No dieter likes being sentenced to nibble on carrots and celery while the rest of the family feasts on heartier fare.

To solve this problem, we've concocted a series of recipes to satisfy the often deprived dieter. Our family-style reducing plan works by a simple system of substitutions and omissions in the kitchen. The dieter will hardly notice the difference. The diet dinner and dessert look every bit as appetizing as the meal for the rest of the family. And because the diet portions taste so good, the satisfied dieter will find that it's much easier to stick to the reducing system.

To carry out this scheme, cooking habits need only minor changes. Remove the dieter's portion from the family pot before adding calorie-laden ingredients. Serve butter, margarine, mayonnaise, and other high-calorie extras from separate containers at the table. Dieters can abstain or if they prefer, they can add their own low-calorie substitutes. Both the dieter and the rest of the family will find all these recipes equally satisfying.

Round Steak Stroganoff

Dieter's version cuts down on calories by eliminating the sour cream and using a measured amount of hot cooked noodles. That's not too much of a sacrifice for a determined dieter.

- 1 pound boneless beef round steak, cut ¾ inch thick and fat trimmed
- 1 tablespoon cornstarch
- ½ teaspoon salt
- 1¼ cups water
- 1 tablespoon tomato paste
- 1½ teaspoons instant beef bouillon granules
- 2 tablespoons diet imitation margarine
- 1 2½-ounce can sliced mushrooms, drained
- ½ cup shredded carrot
- ½ cup chopped onion
- 1 clove garlic, minced
- 1 tablespoon cornstarch
- 2 tablespoons dry red wine
- ½ cup dairy sour cream
- 2¾ cups hot, cooked noodles

Partially freeze the beef round steak; slice thinly into bite-size strips. Combine 1 tablespoon cornstarch and salt. Coat the beef strips with the cornstarch mixture; set aside. In small bowl combine water, tomato paste, and instant beef bouillon granules, set aside.

In skillet brown meat in diet imitation margarine. Push the meat to one side of skillet; add the drained mushrooms, carrot, onion, and garlic. Cook 2 to 3 minutes or till tender. Blend in the remaining 1 tablespoon cornstarch. Add the tomato paste mixture. Cook and stir till mixture is thickened and bubbly. Stir in the dry red wine.

Reserve ¾ *cup* of the beef-vegetable mixture for the dieter; keep warm. Stir sour cream into the remaining beef-vegetable mixture; heat through (do not boil). Reserve ½ cup of the hot, cooked noodles for dieter. Serve the remaining noodles with sour cream-beef mixture. Makes 3 regular servings and 1 diet serving. One diet serving (¾ cup beef-vegetable mixture and ½ cup noodles) equals:

- 3 Lean Meat Exchanges
- 1 Bread Exchange
- 1 Vegetable Exchange
- ½ Fat Exchange

Cranberry-Orange Chicken

Dieter abstains from chicken skin and browning.

- 1 3-pound broiler-fryer chicken, cut up
- 1 10½-ounce can *condensed* beef broth
- ¾ cup low-calorie cranberry juice cocktail
- 2 tablespoons butter *or* margarine
- 2 medium oranges, thinly sliced
- 1 tablespoon cornstarch

Combine chicken neck, giblets, and condensed beef broth. Simmer, covered, 1 hour; strain. Add cranberry juice to broth; boil till reduced to 1 cup. Skin and halve chicken breast lengthwise; place in small baking dish. Sprinkle with *salt;* cover. Brown remaining chicken in butter or margarine; place in 11x7½x2-inch baking dish. Sprinkle with *salt.* Bake chicken, covered, in 350° oven 40 minutes. Top breast with ¼ of the orange slices. Top remaining chicken with remaining orange slices. Bake, uncovered, 10 minutes more. Blend cornstarch into 1 tablespoon cold *water;* stir into broth mixture. Cook and stir till thickened. Top breast with ¼ *cup* of the sauce. Pass remaining sauce. Makes 3 regular servings and 1 diet serving. One diet serving (1 breast and ¼ cup sauce) equals:

- 3½ Lean Meat Exchanges
- 1 Fruit Exchange

Tropical Fruit Cup

Coconut and brown sugar are taboo for the dieter.

- 1 20-ounce can pineapple chunks (juice pack)
- 2 medium oranges, peeled and sliced
- 1½ cups seedless green grapes
- ½ cup shredded coconut
- 6 ounces neufchatel cheese, softened
- 2 tablespoons brown sugar

Drain pineapple; reserve ⅓ cup juice. Halve orange slices. Combine fruits; reserve ½ *cup* for dieter. Add coconut to remainder. Chill fruit. Combine cheese and reserved juice. Spoon *1 tablespoon* of the cheese mixture atop dieter's portion. Stir brown sugar into remaining cheese mixture; spoon atop fruit-coconut mixture. Makes 4 regular servings and 1 diet serving. One diet serving (1 fruit cup) equals:

- ½ Lean Meat Exchange
- 1½ Fruit Exchanges
- ¼ Fat Exchange

Shrimp Mélange

Dieter swaps an aromatic wine sauce for the rich cheese sauce and sidesteps the crumb topping for a dash of paprika.

- 1 **pound fresh *or* frozen shelled shrimp**
- 1 **9-ounce package frozen artichoke hearts**
- 5 **teaspoons cornstarch**
- ½ **teaspoon salt**
- ½ **teaspoon paprika**
- 1⅔ **cups skim milk**
- ¼ **cup dry white wine**
- ¾ **cup shredded Swiss cheese (3 ounces)**
- 2¼ **cups cooked rice**
- ⅛ **teaspoon dried basil, crushed**
- ⅛ **teaspoon dried oregano, crushed**
  Paprika
- 1 **tablespoon butter *or* margarine, melted**
- 3 **tablespoons fine dry bread crumbs**

Thaw shrimp, if frozen. Prepare artichokes according to package directions; set aside. In medium saucepan combine cornstarch, salt, ½ teaspoon paprika, and dash *pepper*. Gradually stir in skim milk. Cook and stir till mixture is thickened and bubbly. Stir in wine; heat through. Reserve ½ *cup* of the sauce for dieter. Stir Swiss cheese into remaining sauce; cook and stir till cheese melts. Set aside. Combine rice, basil, and oregano. Place ¼ *cup* of the rice mixture in bottom of a 10-ounce casserole for dieter. Place remaining rice in 1-quart casserole.

Drop shrimp in 3 cups boiling salted *water;* reduce heat and simmer gently 1 to 3 minutes or till shrimp turn pink. Drain. Combine shrimp and artichokes. Top dieter's rice mixture with ¾ *cup* shrimp-artichoke mixture and the ½ cup reserved sauce. Top large casserole with remaining shrimp-artichoke mixture and cheese sauce. Sprinkle both dishes with additional paprika. Combine butter or margarine with bread crumbs; sprinkle atop large casserole. Bake large casserole in 350° oven 10 minutes. Place small casserole in oven; bake both casseroles 20 to 25 minutes more. Makes 4 regular servings and 1 diet serving. One diet serving (1 individual casserole) equals:

● ● ● 3 Lean Meat Exchanges

◖ ½ Bread Exchange

● 1 Vegetable Exchange

◖ ½ Milk Exchange

Spinach-Topped Halibut

Includes just enough of the rich cheese sauce to make the dieter's entrée special.

- 1½ **pounds fresh *or* frozen halibut steaks**
- 4 **cups water**
- ⅓ **cup lemon juice**
- 1 **small onion, sliced and separated into rings**
- ¼ **cup chopped celery**
- ¼ **teaspoon salt**
- ⅛ **teaspoon freshly ground pepper**
- 1 **10-ounce package frozen chopped spinach**
- ¼ **teaspoon ground nutmeg**
- 1 **1¼-ounce envelope cheese sauce mix**
- 1 **cup skim milk**
  Lemon wedges

Thaw fish, if frozen. In 12-inch skillet combine water, lemon juice, onion, celery, salt, and pepper. Bring to boil; simmer 5 minutes. Add halibut; simmer, covered, 5 to 10 minutes or till fish flakes easily with a fork. Carefully remove fish to 13x9x2-inch baking pan.

Meanwhile, cook spinach according to package directions; drain and stir in nutmeg. Reserve ¼ *cup* of the spinach mixture for dieter. Prepare cheese sauce mix according to package directions *except* use the skim milk instead of whole milk. Spoon *1 tablespoon* of the cheese sauce into dieter's spinach mixture; spread atop *1* of the halibut steaks. Combine remaining cheese sauce and spinach; spread atop remaining steaks for regular servings. Broil all halibut portions 4 to 5 inches from heat 2 to 3 minutes. Serve all halibut portions with lemon wedges. Makes 3 regular servings and 1 diet serving. One diet serving (1 halibut steak and ¼ cup spinach mixture) equals:

● ● ● ● 4 Lean Meat Exchanges

● 1 Vegetable Exchange

◖ ½ Fat Exchange

Shrimp Melange: Family's portion, top right, and dieter's portion, bottom left.

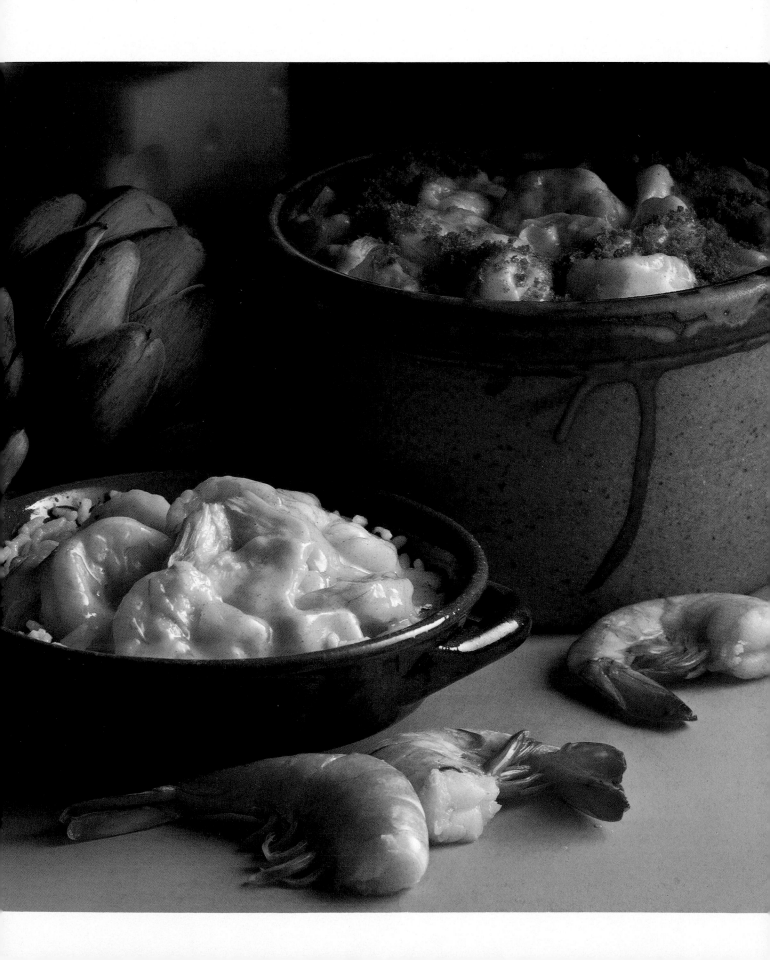

eating out

Eating out doesn't have to mean eating too much. In fact, you can overcome the temptations confronted when eating out by using the Food Exchange formula. Whether it's a cozy dinner with friends or a gala restaurant affair, the dieting tactics you use are found in the Food Exchange system.

Because the Food Exchange Meal Plans in this book fit into normal eating patterns, it's no trick at all to eat out and enjoy it. A night out for an occasional rest from the cooking routine is good for everyone. Even the reducer can enjoy eating out without breaking the diet and going off the Daily Meal Plan.

Restaurant tips

Serious dieters choose their restaurants wisely. They look for restaurants with a variety of menu items and search out those that specialize in lighter entrées. That way, the dieters *and* the non-dieters in the crowd can select what they want.

Some Oriental restaurants feature foods that are well-suited for the dieter. Their low-calorie vegetable dishes and low-fat stir-frying techniques are an appealing combination. In French restaurants, the nouvelle cuisine, a lighter style of cooking, is slowly taking the place of the calorie-laden cuisine that has been dominant. With the Food Exchanges as your guide, it's easy to enjoy many of the gourmet restaurants and still lose weight.

Occasionally, you may want to choose a restaurant noted for its salad bar. You'll find that making a meal out of greens and garnishes is a dining adventure your waistline can afford. Usually you'll be able to round out the salad meal with a steaming soup and a slice of bread. Sometimes you'll find yourself in a traditional restaurant with an unimaginative menu. Don't make a fuss and ask for impossible food items not listed on the menu. Flexibility is the key. Remember: No one's going to force you to clean your plate. You can always ask for a "doggy bag" to carry home the leftovers.

Try ordering a hearty meat or seafood appetizer rather than a main dish and then make a meal out of salad, bread, vegetable, and the appetizer. You'll discover that a restaurant meal of this type can be easily adapted to meet the Exchange requirements of any of the Daily Meal Plans.

Diner's choice

Usually a first-rate diet meal can be assembled at most restaurants if you know how.

Before dinner

High calorie, low-nutrient before-dinner drinks and cocktails send your diet astray faster than any other food, and they stimulate your appetite. Make dinner reservations; arrive on time so you won't be forced to wait in the cocktail lounge, drinking calories to kill time.

There are several alternatives to the "What do you want to drink?" question. Choose a low-calorie soft drink, a glass of carbonated water on the rocks, or try the popular bottled mineral waters with a twist of lime as a garnish—they all qualify as Free Exchanges. For a nutritive punch, select orange juice and count it as a dinnertime Fruit Exchange.

If you can't avoid a wait in the cocktail lounge, choose your seat far from the cocktail nibbles. It doesn't take long to spoil dinner and your diet with "a few bites" of cheese and crackers or nuts. If it's just not possible to resist the temptation, remember the Food Exchanges. For example, 20 Spanish peanuts equal one Fat Exchange while one ounce of cheddar cheese equals one High-Fat Meat Exchange. If possible, opt for the raw vegetable relishes. They pack a less potent caloric punch.

Spend an Exchange on the first course if you have one to spare. Remember that nonfat bouillon and consommé are free. Melon in season, fresh fruit cups, and fruit juices are refreshing appetizer offerings that count as Fruit Exchanges. Seafood appetizers count as Meat Exchanges, while tomato or vegetable juice cocktails are tallied as Vegetable Exchanges. Be leery of heavy, creamed soups such as cream of mushroom or potato. They add unwanted Exchanges. Avoid fried appetizers, because they usually contribute more than their fair share of fat.

Restaurants often serve a basket of bread with butter. This will no doubt tempt you during the minutes before the main course arrives, so beware. Take one roll and one pat of butter to last the whole meal, *or* exhibit a show of will power and pass up the bread and butter completely.

Dinner

With the Food Exchanges as your guide, you can easily navigate your way through the main courses of any menu. Order broiled or baked poultry, fish, or lean meat. By all means, avoid fried foods. Serving sizes are usually larger than your Exchange allotment. If they are, don't eat the entire portion. Take the remaining food home so you can use it in a salad or sandwich the next day. Eat around the breading, fat, rich sauces, gravies, or stuffings that may accompany your main dish.

When ordering vegetables, your Food Exchange expertise should shine. If you order a baked potato, ask for butter or sour cream separately so you can control the amount you add. One small baked potato counts as one Bread Exchange, while one teaspoon of butter or two tablespoons dairy sour cream count as one Fat Exchange. Many restaurants now feature rice, another member of the Bread Exchange family and certainly a wiser choice than fat-laden French fries or hash browns. But if you can't resist French fries, there's no need to deprive yourself. Just be sure to subtract one Bread Exchange and one Fat Exchange for every eight fries. Consider a double portion of carrots, broccoli, or whatever vegetable the restaurant has to offer, as long as your daily allotment of Food Exchanges allows it.

A number of salad greens (chicory, Chinese cabbage, endive, escarole, lettuce, parsley, and watercress) are Free Exchanges and can be eaten in any amount. Vegetables such as celery, cucumber, mushrooms, onions, and tomatoes add one Exchange per one-half cup serving. Radishes are free. When it comes to dressing for your salad, it's best to carry along your favorite brand of low-calorie dressing. If that's too much trouble, go without or ask for vinegar and oil (a very light touch on the oil, please—one teaspoon counts as one Fat Exchange and packs 45 calories). One tablespoon of regular French dressing or Italian dressing counts as one Fat Exchange.

After dinner

In the dessert department, you're in luck if fresh or baked fruit is listed on the menu. If there aren't any suitable choices, order a cup of steaming coffee or tea and sip it slowly.

Remember the handy clip-out Food Exchanges on pages 89-92. When you eat out, carry these condensed lists with you for reference. Besides the Food Exchange Lists and the Daily Meal Plans, Exchange information for many of the national restaurant chains is included. By consulting this information, you can have a bite at any of these restaurants without feeling guilty.

Sample menu selections

Let us take you through the sample menu on the following page and point out the maneuvers we've used to trim corners. Using the Food Exchange framework, we've adjusted many of the menu offerings to meet your reducing requirements. Although you can't eat everything offered on the menu, you have plenty of choices.

restaurant menus

dinner

APPETIZERS

Fruit cup with sherbet*
Prosciutto with melon*
French-fried mushrooms

Gulf shrimp cocktail*
Blue point oysters on
   the half shell*

CHEF'S SPECIALTIES

New York strip steak*
Roast prime rib of beef*
Beef en brochette*
Rock Cornish hen with
   wild rice stuffing*
Creamy chicken crepes

Broiled lobster tail
   with lemon butter*
Batter-fried shrimp
Crab-stuffed flounder
Catch of the day*
Lamb with mint jelly*

VEGETABLES

Steamed fresh
   asparagus*
Fresh garden peas*

Baked Idaho potato*
Hash brown potatoes
Rice pilaf*

SALADS

Bouquet of fresh fruit*
Green garden salad*

Fresh spinach salad
   with bacon dressing*

DESSERTS

French apple tart
Spicy baked peaches*
Cheesecake

Chocolate mousse
Strawberries and
   cream*

BEVERAGES

Coffee*
Tea*

Milk*
Soft drinks

Dining out can be fun using the Food Exchange formula. Select foods within limits of your Daily Meal Plan.

Order a fruit cup; leave the sherbet. Count prosciutto as a High-Fat Meat. Order oysters or shrimp; use lemon instead of cocktail sauce.

Main dish servings are typically larger than Exchange allotments. Take leftovers home. Order lobster without lemon butter; add fresh lemon instead. Order the "catch" if it's baked or broiled. Order lamb; leave the jelly.

Request asparagus or peas without butter or sauces. Ditto for baked potato—add your own. Estimate serving sizes carefully.

Go easy on the salad dressing. Order spinach salad without bacon dressing; try lemon juice instead.

Ask whether peaches are prepared with sugar. Ask for strawberries and cream separately; add cream sparingly.

Coffee and tea are free. Milk is allowed, but avoid the soft drinks unless low-cal brands are available.

*possible menu selections

restaurant exchanges

Are you just dying for that forbidden slice of pizza? Does a thick milkshake sound too good to pass up? Or does your busy schedule mean you often grab a quick bite at a fast-food restaurant? Whatever your reason, you can enjoy the convenience of eating out at selected restaurants and know exactly how your meal stacks up in terms of Food Exchanges. Clip out this handy guide and carry it with you as a quick reference.

Restaurant and foods	Serving size	Exchanges per serving
McDonald's®		
hamburger	1	1 lean meat + 2 bread + 1 fat
cheeseburger	1	1½ lean meat + 2 bread + 1½ fat
Quarter Pounder® (wt. before cooking 4 oz. [113.4 gr.])	1	3 lean meat + 2 bread + 3 fat
Quarter Pounder® with cheese	1	4 lean meat + 2 bread + 4 fat
Big Mac™	1	3 lean meat + 2½ bread + 4½ fat
Filet-O-Fish™	1	1½ lean meat + 2½ bread + 3½ fat
French fries (regular size)	1 serving	1½ bread + 2 fat
Egg McMuffin®	1	2 lean meat + 1½ bread + 3 fat
scrambled eggs	1 serving	1½ lean meat + 1¾ fat
hot cakes with butter and syrup	1 serving	4 bread + 3 fruit + 2 fat
chocolate shake	1	3½ bread + ½ milk + 2 fat
vanilla shake	1	3 bread + ½ milk + 2 fat
Burger King®		
hamburger	1	2 lean meat + 2 bread + 1½ fat
hamburger with cheese	1	2 lean meat + 2 bread + 2½ fat
Whopper® sandwich	1	3 lean meat + 3½ bread + 5½ fat
Whopper Jr.® sandwich	1	1½ lean meat + 2 bread + 3 fat
Whaler® sandwich	1	3 lean meat + 3½ bread + 5½ fat
onion rings (regular size)	1 serving	1½ bread + ½ vegetable + 2½ fat

Restaurant and foods	Serving size	Exchanges per serving
Hardee's®		
hamburger	1	2 lean meat + 2 bread + 1½ fat
cheeseburger	1	2 lean meat + 2 bread + 2 fat
double cheeseburger	1	3½ lean meat + 2 bread + 4 fat
Big Deluxe™	1	3½ lean meat + 3 bread + 6 fat
Big Twin®	1	3 lean meat + 2 bread + 3 fat
fish sandwich	1	1½ lean meat + 3 bread + 4 fat
hot dog	1	1 lean meat + 1½ bread + 4 fat
roast beef sandwich	1	1½ lean meat + 3 bread + 2 fat
French fries (small size)	1 serving	2 bread + 2½ fat
apple turnover	1	1 bread + 2 fruit + 3 fat
milkshake	1	3½ bread + ½ milk + 2 fat
Sizzler Family Steak House®		
lo-cal platter	1	4 lean meat + 2 bread + 1½ fat
high protein platter	1	8 lean meat + 2 bread + 3 fat
Arthur Treacher's		
fish	2 pieces	2 lean meat + 1½ bread + 3 fat
chicken	2 pieces	3½ lean meat + 1 bread + 2½ fat
shrimp	7 pieces	1½ lean meat + 2 bread + 3½ fat
chips	1 serving	2 bread + 3 fat
cole slaw	1 serving	2 vegetable + 1½ fat
fish sandwich	1	1½ lean meat + 2½ bread + 3 fat
chicken sandwich	1	1½ lean meat + 3 bread + 3 fat
Pizza Hut®		
Thin 'N Crispy® pizza (13-inch diameter):		
standard cheese	2 slices	2 lean meat + 3 bread + ½ fat
SuperStyle cheese	2 slices	3 lean meat + 3 bread + 1 fat
standard pepperoni	2 slices	2 lean meat + 3 bread + 1½ fat
SuperStyle pepperoni	2 slices	2½ lean meat + 3 bread + 2 fat
standard pork and mushroom	2 slices	2 lean meat + 3 bread + 1½ fat
SuperStyle pork and mushroom	2 slices	3 lean meat + 3 bread + 2 fat
Supreme	2 slices	2 lean meat + 3 bread + 2 fat
Super Supreme	2 slices	3 lean meat + 3 bread + 3 fat

food exchange lists

meat

LEAN MEAT EXCHANGE

Each serving below is based on cooked meat with fat trimmed. One Exchange provides seven grams protein, three grams fat, and 55 calories. Most Exchanges except shellfish are fairly low in saturated fat and cholesterol.

beef: 1 ounce — dried beef, flank steak, sirloin, tenderloin, chuck, plate spareribs, plate short ribs, round, bottom or top, plate skirt steak, all cuts rump

lamb: 1 ounce — shank, leg, rib, shoulder, sirloin, loin

pork: 1 ounce — leg (whole rump, center shank), fully cooked ham (center slices)

veal: 1 ounce — leg, shoulder, loin, cutlets, rib, shank

fish: any fresh, canned, or frozen 1 ounce — bass, sea or striped, carp, catfish, cod, eel, flounder, haddock, hake, halibut, herring, lake or Atlantic, mackerel, mullet, pike, pollock, pompano, red snapper, rockfish, salmon, sardines, smelt, sole, swordfish, tuna, whitefish, perch, clams, crab, oysters, scallops, shrimp, lobster

poultry: without skin 1 ounce — Cornish hen, turkey, pheasant, chicken, Guinea hen

cheeses containing less than 5% butterfat 1 ounce

cottage cheese, dry and 2% butterfat ¼ cup

dried beans and peas (omit 1 Bread Exchange) ½ cup cooked

MEDIUM-FAT MEAT EXCHANGE

Each serving is based on cooked meat and counts as one Medium-Fat Meat Exchange. Because of their higher fat content, Medium-Fat Meat Exchanges count as one Lean Meat Exchange and one-half Fat Exchange on the Daily Meal Plans. One Medium-Fat Meat Exchange supplies seven grams protein, five and one-half grams fat, and 75 calories. Only peanut butter is low in saturated fat and cholesterol.

beef: 1 ounce — ground beef (15% fat), ground round (commercial), corned beef (canned), rib eye steak

pork: 1 ounce — loin (all cuts tenderloin), shoulder arm, picnic, shoulder blade, Boston roast, Canadian-style bacon

variety meat — beef, veal, pork, or lamb: 1 ounce (high in cholesterol) — heart, liver, sweetbreads, kidney

cheese: 1 ounce — mozzarella, ricotta 1 ounce, parmesan 3 tbsp., farmer's cheese, neufchatel 1 ounce

cottage cheese, creamed ¼ cup

egg (high in cholesterol) 1

peanut butter (omit 2 additional Fat Exchanges) 2 tbsp.

HIGH-FAT MEAT EXCHANGE

Each serving below is based on cooked meat and counts as one High-Fat Meat Exchange. Because of their high fat content, foods in this Exchange List count as one Lean Meat Exchange and one Fat Exchange. One High-Fat Meat Exchange supplies seven grams of protein, eight grams of fat, and 100 calories.

beef: 1 ounce — brisket, corned beef brisket, ground beef (more than 20% fat), hamburger (commercial), ground chuck (commercial), rib roast, rib steak, top loin steak

lamb: 1 ounce — breast

veal: 1 ounce — breast

pork: 1 ounce — spareribs, loin back ribs, ground pork, deviled ham, cook-before-eating ham (country-style)

poultry: 1 ounce — capon, duck (domestic), goose

cheese: cheddar types 1 ounce

cold cuts 4½ x ⅛-inch slice

frankfurter 1 small

fruit

The amount of each fruit listed (with no sugar added) counts as one Fruit Exchange. Fruits are nonfat. One Exchange contains 10 grams carbohydrate and 40 calories.

apple	1 small	figs, fresh or dried	1	orange juice	½ cup
apple juice or cider	⅓ cup	grapefruit	½	papaya	¾ cup
applesauce (unsweetened)	½ cup	grapefruit juice	½ cup	peach	1 medium
apricots, fresh	2 medium	grapes	12	pear	1 small
apricots, dried	4 halves	grape juice	¼ cup	persimmon, native	1 medium
banana	½ small	mango	½ small	pineapple	½ cup
berries		melon		pineapple juice	⅓ cup
strawberries	¾ cup	cantaloupe	¼ small	plums	2 medium
other berries	½ cup	honeydew	⅛ medium	prunes	2 medium
cherries	10 large	watermelon	1 cup	prune juice	¼ cup
cranberries	as desired	nectarine	1 small	raisins	2 tbsp.
dates	2	orange	1 small	tangerine	1 medium

vegetable

Each half-cup serving counts as one Exchange and provides two grams protein, five grams carbohydrate, and 25 calories. Vegetables are nonfat. Free vegetables are listed below and in the Free List.

asparagus	eggplant	rutabaga
beans, green or yellow	mushrooms	sauerkraut
bean sprouts	okra	spinach and other greens
beets	onions	summer squash
broccoli	peppers	tomatoes
brussels sprouts	rhubarb	tomato juice
cabbage		turnips
carrots		vegetable juice cocktail
caul flower		zucchini
celery		
cucumbers		

The following raw vegetables are all Free Exchanges and may be eaten in any amounts:

chicory	radishes
Chinese cabbage	watercress
endive	
escarole	
lettuce	
parsley	

milk

Milk Exchanges are shown below. Lowfat and whole milk products cost extra Fat Exchanges. One Exchange equals eight grams protein, 12 grams carbohydrate, and 80 calories.

nonfat fortified milk:

skim or nonfat milk	1 cup	canned evaporated skim milk	½ cup
nonfat dry milk powder	⅓ cup	buttermilk, made from skim milk	1 cup
yogurt, made from skim milk (plain)	1 cup		

lowfat fortified milk:

1% fat milk (omit ½ Fat Exchange)	1 cup	yogurt, made from 2% milk (plain) (omit 1 Fat Exchange)	¾ cup
2% fat milk (omit 1 Fat Exchange)	1 cup		

whole milk (omit 2 Fat Exchanges):

whole milk	1 cup	canned evaporated whole milk	½ cup
yogurt, made from whole milk (plain)	1 cup	buttermilk, made from whole milk	1 cup

bread

Each serving of the following breads, cereals, crackers, dried beans, starchy vegetables, and prepared foods counts as one Bread Exchange. All items except those listed as prepared foods are lowfat. Be sure to charge yourself for the extra Fat Exchanges contained in the prepared foods. One Bread Exchange provides two grams of protein, 15 grams of carbohydrate, and 70 calories.

bread:

white, whole wheat, French, Italian, rye, pumpernickel, or raisin	1 slice	hamburger bun	½
bagel, small	½	dried bread crumbs	3 tbsp.
English muffin, small	½	tortilla, 6 inch	1
plain dinner roll	1		
frankfurter bun	½		

cereal:

bran flakes	½ cup	popcorn (popped, no fat added)	3 cups
other ready-to-eat unsweetened cereal	¾ cup	cornmeal (dry)	2 tbsp.
puffed cereal (unfrosted)	1 cup	flour	2½ tbsp.
cooked cereal	½ cup	wheat germ	¼ cup
cooked grits	½ cup		
cooked rice or barley	½ cup		
cooked pasta, macaroni, or noodles	½ cup		

crackers:

arrowroot	3	pretzels, 3⅛x⅛ inch	25
graham, 2½ inch	2	rye wafers, 3½x2 inch	3
matzo, 6x4 inch	½	saltines	6
oyster	20	soda, 2½-inch square	4

beans, peas, and lentils:

beans, peas, lentils (dried, cooked) (omit 1 Lean Meat Exchange)	½ cup	baked beans, no pork (canned)	¼ cup

starchy vegetables:

corn	⅓ cup	pumpkin	¾ cup
corn on cob	1 small	winter squash	½ cup
lima beans	½ cup	yam or sweet potato	¼ cup
parsnips	⅔ cup		
peas (canned or frozen)	½ cup		
potato (white)	1 small		
potato (mashed)	½ cup		

prepared foods:

muffin, plain small (omit 1 Fat Exchange)	1	potato or corn chips (omit 2 Fat Exchanges)	15
pancake, 5x½ inch (omit 1 Fat Exchange)	1	corn muffin, 2 inch (omit 1 Fat Exchange)	1
corn bread, 2x2x1 inch (omit 1 Fat Exchange)	1	crackers, round butter type (omit 1 Fat Exchange)	5
biscuit, 2-inch diameter (omit 1 Fat Exchange)	1		
potatoes, French-fried (omit 1 Fat Exchange)	8		
waffle, 5x½ inch (omit 1 Fat Exchange)	1		

fat

Fats below are designated as saturated, monounsaturated, or polyunsaturated. Saturated fats are found primarily in animal food products and are believed to raise the level of cholesterol in the blood, a risk factor associated with heart disease. Heart specialists recommend substituting the unsaturated fats for the saturated fats in the diet whenever possible. Vegetable oils such as corn, cottonseed, safflower, soybean, and sunflower are low in saturated fats. The fats listed below are saturated unless marked with an asterisk (*). One asterisk (*) indicates a fat content that is primarily monounsaturated. Two asterisks (**) indicate a fat content that is primarily polyunsaturated, while three asterisks (***) indicate a polyunsaturated fat content only if the product is made with corn, cottonseed, safflower, soy, or sunflower oil. One Fat Exchange provides five grams of fat and 45 calories.

avocado* (4-inch diameter)	⅛	margarine, regular	1 tsp.
bacon, crisp-cooked	1 slice	lard	1 tsp.
bacon fat	1 tsp.	mayonnaise***	1 tsp.
butter	1 tsp.	olives*	5 small
cream cheese	1 tbsp.	salad dressing***	2 tsp.
cream, light	2 tbsp.	mayonnaise- type	
cream, sour	2 tbsp.	salt pork	¾-in. cube
cream, whipping	1 tbsp.		
dressing, Italian salad***	1 tbsp.	mayonnaise-***	2 tsp.
dressing, French salad***	1 tbsp.		
margarine,*** soft (tub or stick)	1 tsp.		

nuts:

almonds*	10 whole	walnuts**	6 small
pecans*	2 large	other*	6 small
	peanuts* Spanish	20 whole	
	Virginia	10 whole	

oil:

1 tsp.	corn** cottonseed**	safflower** soy**	sunflower** olive*	peanut*

free

Listed below are flavor bonuses with Free Exchange ratings. Also included on this list are raw vegetables which can be eaten in any amount desired.

salt	low-calorie carbonated beverages	unflavored gelatin unsweetened	endive escarole
pepper			
herbs			lettuce
spices	low-calorie flavored gelatin	pickles	parsley
coffee		chicory	radishes
tea			watercress
lemon		Chinese cabbage	
lime			
vinegar			
mustard			
nonfat bouillon			
non-caloric sweetener			
horseradish			

Food Exchange Lists (pages 26-30) are based on material in the booklet *Exchange Lists for Meal Planning* prepared by committees of the American Diabetes Association, Inc. and the American Dietetic Association.

daily meal plans

FOOD EXCHANGES AND COLOR SYMBOLS

		1,000 cal. per day no. of Exchanges	1,200 cal. per day no. of Exchanges	1,500 cal. per day no. of Exchanges
breakfast	Lean Meat Exchange	1	1	2
	Bread Exchange	1	1	2
	Fruit Exchange	1	1	1
	Milk Exchange	½	½	½
	Fat Exchange	1	2	2
	Free Exchange	as desired	as desired	as desired
lunch	Lean Meat Exchange	2	2	2
	Bread Exchange	1	1	2
	Fruit Exchange	1	1	1
	Vegetable Exchange	1	2	2
	Milk Exchange	1	1	1
	Fat Exchange	1	1	2
	Free Exchange	as desired	as desired	as desired
dinner	Lean Meat Exchange	2	4	4
	Bread Exchange	1	1	1
	Fruit Exchange	1	1	1
	Vegetable Exchange	1	2	2
	Milk Exchange	½	½	½
	Fat Exchange	2	2	3
	Free Exchange	as desired	as desired	as desired

Planning diet menus isn't difficult if you use the Food Exchanges to guide you. Choose a meal plan giving a daily calorie deficit that lets you reduce no more than two pounds a week (see pages 9-11). Follow the food allotments in your Daily Meal Plan and make menu selections from the Food Exchange Lists (see pages 26-35) and the recipe section.

sack lunches

Brown-bagging it

Lunch sometimes must be portable, stowed in a brown bag, a lunch box, or even an attaché case. Don't let this limit your lunchtime creativity or cramp your reducing style. A brown-bag lunch can be appetizing and make a contribution to your weight loss program.

Mainstay sandwiches

A hearty sandwich is the traditional foundation of a brown-bag lunch. Weight watchers, too, can lunch on sandwiches.

Sandwich construction begins with bread. Choices include white, whole wheat, Italian, French, rye, pumpernickel, and raisin. English muffins, hamburger buns, and bagels are also suitable.

If you're following the 1,000- or 1,200-calorie Daily Meal Plans, you may wish to transfer one Bread Exchange from breakfast or dinner to lunch to allow two slices of bread for a sandwich. If not, try stretching the lunchtime allotment of one Bread Exchange in one of two ways. You can use very thin bread (white or whole wheat). Two slices count as one Bread Exchange. Or you can pack sandwich ingredients separately and assemble an open-faced sandwich at lunchtime.

Spread your choice of bread with mustard, diet imitation margarine, or low-calorie salad dressing substitute. Next, layer meat slices atop. Meats listed in the Lean Meat Exchanges are the best choices because they conserve fat for other uses. Cooked chicken, turkey, ham (center-cut, not boiled) and lean roast beef are possible selections that cost you no extra fat. Boiled ham and cooked pork are Medium-Fat Meat Exchanges, while most common cold cuts are High-Fat Meat Exchanges.

Team your meat selection with a slice of cheese. One ounce of most cheddar types counts as one High-Fat Meat Exchange. Trim Fat Exchanges by selecting low-calorie process cheese product. A one-ounce serving equals one Lean Meat Exchange. For a change of pace, try scrambled eggs or egg salad as sandwich fillers. Don't forget about canned foods such as tuna, chicken, salmon, ham, and shrimp for sandwich makings.

Lettuce adds crunch and freshness to a sandwich without adding extra Exchanges. Bean sprouts and slices of cucumber, green pepper, or onion are crisp sandwich ingredients, and they cost only one Vegetable Exchange per one-half cup.

Sandwiches cannot be stored without refrigeration for long periods of time. If they must stand at room temperature, freeze them overnight. Remove from the freezer on your way to work and they'll be thawed by lunchtime.

Sandwich substitutes

Salads provide a tasty alternative to sandwiches. If refrigerator space is available, use it to store perishables. Otherwise use a wide-mouth thermos. Take along chicken, tuna, egg, or ham salad and pack lettuce and tomato separately. Assemble the salad quickly at lunchtime. For variety, pack a chef's salad, cottage cheese, or your favorite yogurt. You'll appreciate the versatility a thermos (or refrigerator) allows.

You also can use a thermos to keep soup, chowder, chili, or stew piping hot. Pack a thick slice of crusty French bread, too.

Sandwich supplements

Round out the sack lunch with suitable supplements. Fruit is a logical choice. Apples, oranges, bananas, plums, and pears all pack well. Or you can carry chilled canned fruit in a wide-mouth thermos. Cans of fruit juice can be frozen the night before and removed from the freezer in the morning. Juice will be thawed by lunchtime but still frosty. Vegetable relishes add a crisp accent. Dill pickles add tang and they're free.

how to stay slim

After you've trimmed down to your ideal weight, try to maintain it. Food Exchanges make it easier, but staying slim requires a lifetime commitment. Remember that it's much easier to gain unwanted pounds than it is to lose them. Don't let extra pounds creep up on you. Learn how to stay slim using the Food Exchange system to guide your eating habits.

Using Food Exchanges to maintain weight

As you approach your dietary goal and are shedding those last few unwanted pounds, think about your maintenance tactics. How are you going to stay slim? Everything you've learned about Food Exchanges, plus the food habits you've acquired, apply to staying slim forever.

Food Exchanges provide a workable and reliable framework for diet maintenance. Follow the 1,500-calorie Daily Meal Plan (page 36), then add your favorite Exchanges to raise your calorie consumption to maintenance levels. Calculate the number of calories necessary to maintain your desirable or ideal weight according to directions on page 10.

Someone whose desirable weight is 100 pounds could follow the 1,500-calorie Daily Meal Plan exactly. The person whose desirable weight is 130 pounds must add enough Exchanges to the 1,500-calorie Daily Meal Plan to add 450 calories. You'll find the calorie values of the various Exchange groups listed on pages 26-30. When adding extra Food Exchanges to the Daily Meal Plan, you will keep the same balance of good nutrition by adding proportionate amounts of the seven Exchanges. It's often as simple as increasing the size of your serving. For example, you could eat a six-ounce sirloin steak instead of a four-ounce steak. This adds two extra ounces of lean meat or two Lean Meat Exchanges. That's 110 additional calories, about one-fourth the amount a 130-pound person needs to increase the 1,500-calorie diet to maintenance levels. You'll find that it's simple to add those maintenance calories. Capitalize on wholesome foods in your diet.

Follow these rules to stay slim:
1. Follow the 1,500-calorie Daily Meal Plan.
2. Add only those Exchanges needed to add calories to maintenance levels.
3. Weigh once a week and cut back on calories if your weight creeps up a few pounds.
4. Exercise regularly.

index

Have BETTER HOMES AND GAR-
DENS® magazine delivered to your
door. For information, write to: MR.
ROBERT AUSTIN, P.O. BOX 4536,
DES MOINES, IA 50336.